Comments and Reviews about Quick & Healthy

D1314376

Recommended in *O, The Oprah Magazine.*

"Ponichtera knows what works in America's kitchen and she's proved it not once but twice." –*Evening Leader*

"My patients love cooking with this cookbook! The delicious, fun recipes are truly quick and healthy, and the nutrition tips are helpful for a lifetime of health. *Quick & Healthy Volume II* is a great addition to any kitchen!" –Georgia Kostas, MPH, RD, Nutrition Director, Cooper Clinic, Dallas, TX, and author of *The Cooper Clinic Solution to the Diet Revolution*

"Her nonfat New York Cheesecake is a true test of one of the book's goals: It tastes great!" – *The Oregonian*

"If saving time and eating healthy is important to you, this is the cookbook for you!" –*Diabetes Balance*

"*Quick & Healthy Volume II* may well become like a Bible for people serious about educating themselves on lower-fat meals that are high on flavor. In a nutshell, Ponichtera has provided a common sense guide and a collection of recipes that are no more than 30% fat." –*Bellevue Leader*

" . . . meets the needs of busy people who say they lack time to cook healthy meals. *Volume II* is filled with healthful and helpful food and nutrition tips, menus and shopping lists, recipes that use common ingredients easily found in the local grocery store, and best of all, recipes for good-tasting family foods that can be prepared in less than 15 minutes." –Nancy Clark, MS, RD, Sports Nutritionist and author of *Nancy Clark's Sports Nutrition Guidebook*

"For those just starting a low-fat lifestyle, or for those veteran health enthusiasts in need of new recipe ideas, *Quick & Healthy Volume II* has something for everyone. *Quick & Healthy Volume II* lives up to its name . . . and then some!" –Peggy Paul, RD, LD, Oregon Dairy Council

"Our customers love *Quick & Healthy Recipes and Ideas* and I know *Volume II* will delight them even more. The recipes are exactly what is claimed by the title–quick and healthy!" –Patty Merrill, Manager of Powell's Books for Cooks

"My favorite cookbooks focused on healthy, quick recipes include the *Quick & Healthy* series by Brenda J. Ponichtera." –David L. Katz, MD, Director of Yale-Griffin Prevention Research Center and medical consultant for ABC News

"Quick and healthy—important for all of us, but of equal importance—tasty and delicious . . . recipes you are sure to enjoy!" —Marion J. Franz, MS, RD, CDE, Director of Nutrition, International Diabetes Center, Minneapolis, MN

"Filled with much useful information for achieving and maintaining a healthy lifestyle. Great recipes. Highly recommended." —John P. Foreyt, PhD, Professor, Department of Medicine, Baylor College of Medicine, and author of *Living Without Dieting*

" . . . she's done it again . . . The recipes are quite doable on a tight schedule and you may just surprise yourself by turning out interesting and varied meals in no time." —*Northwest Walker*

"*Quick & Healthy Volume II* provides a useful collection of convenient recipes using today's available low-fat ingredients." —Lisë Stern, Editor, *The Cookbook Review*

"There are enough recipes and meal ideas to keep you from ever getting bored with those everyday meals, or with preparing them . . . What helps is that the ingredients are all easily obtainable, and the cooking methods are down to earth and as simplified as possible." —*Quick, Easy, Cheap and Simple*

"Ponichtera has succeeded once again in convincing busy people everywhere that you can cook healthy meals quickly and easily." —*The Life Preserver*

". . . it is a must for those who have the first *Quick & Healthy* and are looking for new ideas. The easy-to-prepare recipes are skillfully arranged and clearly written. Also, they have been well tested so one can feel confident they will work." —Sonja L. Connor, MS, RD, Research Associate Professor, and William E. Connor, MD, Professor, Section of Clinical Nutrition, Oregon Health Sciences University; coauthors of *The New American Diet*

"The menus bring palatable dishes together to create quick but healthy meals. The cookbook is the perfect addition to kitchens of folks who are dieting or seeking to maintain their weights." —*The Enquirer-Journal*

"If you prefer eating healthy meals but don't have much time to cook, *Quick & Healthy Volume II* is the cookbook for you." —*Taking Care*

"Ponichtera has combined smart ideas, imagination, and brand name convenience to provide a wealth of good-tasting and good-for-you dishes that are quick and easy to prepare." —*Senior Dynamics*

"The recipes are ones that ordinary people actually could conceive of using in their own kitchens. Both the Spanish Chicken and Seasoned Black Beans were extraordinarily easy and quite flavorful." —*Beaumont Enterprise*

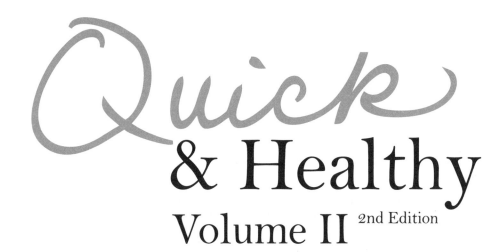

Quick
& Healthy
Volume II ^{2nd Edition}

More help for people who say
they don't have time to cook healthy meals

Brenda J. Ponichtera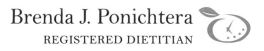
REGISTERED DIETITIAN

ILLUSTRATIONS
Lisa Becharas and Janice Staver

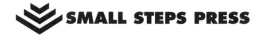 **SMALL STEPS PRESS**

Director, Book Publishing, Robert Anthony; *Managing Editor, Book Publishing,* Abe Ogden; *Production Manager,* Melissa Sprott; *Cover Design,* Vis-à-Vis Creative; *Illustrations,* Lisa Becharas, Janice Staver; *Cover Photography:* Gary Dolgoff; *Printer,* United Graphics, Inc.

Printed in the United States of America
1 3 5 7 9 10 8 6 4 2

Small Steps Press is an imprint of the American Diabetes Association. For information about Small Steps Press or the American Diabetes Association, in English or Spanish, call 1-800-342-2383. To order other Small Steps books, call 1-800-232-6733.

Every effort has been made by the author to include only recipes that have not been previously copyrighted. Should any such published recipe appear in this book, it is without her knowledge and is unintentional. The information and recipes in this book are not intended, nor should anything contained herein be construed, as an attempt to give, or be a substitute for medical advice or medical nutrition therapy. This book is not a medical manual and is not to be used as a substitute for treatment prescribed by your physician.

Consult a health care professional before trying any of the suggestions in this publication. Small Steps Press, ADA, and Brenda Ponichtera assume no responsibility for any injury that may result from the suggestions or information in this publication.

♾ The paper in this publication meets the requirements of the ANSI Standard Z39.48-1992 (permanence of paper).

Small Steps Press titles may be purchased for business or promotional use or for special sales. To purchase bulk copies of this book at a discount, or for custom editions of this book with your logo, contact Small Steps Press at the address below, at booksales@diabetes.org, or by calling 703-299-2046.

For all other inquiries, please call 1-800-342-2383.

Small Steps Press
1701 North Beauregard Street
Alexandria, Virginia 22311

Library of Congress Cataloging-in-Publication Data
Ponichtera, Brenda J.
  Quick & healthy, volume II : more help for people who say they don't have time to cook healthy meals / Brenda J. Ponichtera. -- 2nd ed.
    p. cm.
  Includes bibliographical references and index.
  ISBN 978-0-9816001-1-6 (alk. paper)
  1. Weight loss. 2. Low-cholesterol diet--Recipes. 3. Low-fat diet--Recipes. 4. Diebetes--Diet therapy--Recipes. 5. Quick and easy cookery. I. Title. II. Title: Quick and healthy, volume II.

RM222.2.P625 2009
613.2'5--dc22
                          2008050752

For more information visit http://www.QuickandHealthy.net.

In memory of my father, Walter Niemic.
He would move Heaven for his children.

and

To Ken, Kevin, and Kyle,
my favorite taste testers…and so honest!

Table of Contents

Acknowledgments

Many people helped to make this book a reality, both the first and now the second edition. Thank you to the following for your help and encouragement.

My family for putting up with my hectic schedule. My husband Ken, and sons Kevin and Kyle, ate many a dinner that was a smorgasbord of leftover tested recipes. My sons and their friends also kept me in touch with the reality of teenage appetites.

Nancy Taphouse for playing a key role in recipe testing and computer input.

Friends and artists, Janice Staver and Lisa Becharas, for again sharing their wonderful creativity.

Claudia Schon for her expertise in recipe development and testing.

Recipe testers and recipe contributors: Jana Webb, Yvonne Lorenz, Kay Erickson, Mary Beth Thouvenel, Ellie Timinsky, Evie Wilkinson, Sally Hill, and Beverly Sherrill.

Bruno Amatter and Kate Bass, for providing so many years of support and dedication. I have learned so much from you!

My support at the American Diabetes Association: Rob Anthony, Abe Ogden, Heschel Falek, Melissa Sprott, and Wendy Martin for providing so much help along the way.

The many health professionals who shared their expertise: Julie Conner, RD, PhD, CDN, Madelyn L. Wheeler, MS, RD, CD, CDE, Elizabeth Somer, MA, RD, Connie Evers, MS, RD, Nancy Clark, MS, RD, Bridget Swinney, MS, RD, Monica A. Cengia, MSEd, RD, CDE, Shelie Hartman-Gibbs, RD, Peggy Paul, RD, LD, Jean Farmer, RD, Anne Fletcher, MS, RD, and Tracy Stopler Kasdan, MS, RD.

Photographers Gary Dolgoff and Jim Semlor, for their commitment to excellence.

My fellow Street Walkers, for your miles of support throughout this marathon called Life.

And last but not least, to the many people who used my first book and asked me to write another . . . thank you for your encouragement and enthusiasm.

Preface

Healthful eating doesn't have to take a lot of time in the kitchen. With that in mind, I wrote my first book, *Quick & Healthy Recipes and Ideas*, which is now in its third edition. Since I received many requests for more recipes and menus, I wrote *Quick & Healthy Volume II*. This new second edition of *Volume II* contains even more help for busy households. Besides more simple menus and recipes, included are even more useful tips to help you save time and be healthy. I think you will agree that *Volume II* will be a good addition to anyone's kitchen library.

What is quick? When testing recipes, we decided that quick meant spending less time in the kitchen. Putting together the ingredients for a meal in less than 15 minutes meets that criterion. However, the cooking time can take longer since this does not usually require constant attention.

Fat free or reduced fat? When testing recipes, we compared the flavor using both fat-free and reduced-fat products. Taste is very important if your family is to continue to use a lower-fat product. Keep this in mind when trying new products and find the lower-fat version, whether it be reduced fat or fat free, that your family will enjoy.

If saving time is as important to you as it is to so many, be sure to use the menus and grocery lists. Make copies of the grocery lists, and keep them in a handy place in the kitchen. Encourage family members to add to the list. Keep in mind that shopping once a week, instead of several times a week, is a real time and money saver. You'll also be pleased to know that all of the ingredients used are readily available in most grocery stores.

All of the recipes are low fat and, when combined with other foods for the day, can easily fall within the recommendation of a low-fat diet.

Besides using the recipes in this book, be sure to look at the other helpful sections. If your goal is to eat healthfully and save time, all of the information and recipes in Volume II can help you reach your goal. And remember, if you have children, your example speaks louder than words.

Enjoy in good health.

Brenda J. Ponichtera
Registered Dietitian

Recipe Notes

Sodium

Salt is listed as an optional ingredient in the recipes and is therefore not included in the nutrient analysis of the recipe. When using frozen or canned products, those with no salt added or reduced salt were used. If you are not accustomed to using sodium-reduced products, it may be more acceptable for your family if you make a gradual transition.

Fiber

Recipes that provide significant fiber include one of the following notations:
- For 3–4 grams of fiber—*One serving is a good source of fiber.*
- For 5 or more grams of fiber—*One serving is an excellent source of fiber.*

Fiber Adjustment for Exchanges and Carb Servings

Carb servings and exchanges for the recipes have been adjusted for fiber. If the fiber is more than 5 grams, half of the grams of fiber are subtracted from the total grams of carbohydrate when figuring exchanges and carb servings.

Using Fresh Produce and Saving Time

Fresh produce is used in all recipes unless otherwise listed as frozen or canned. Save money by buying whole vegetables, and save time by cleaning and slicing them all at once. Refrigerate in resealable plastic bags. A salad spinner can make cleaning lettuce a quick task. Also save time by purchasing produce that is cleaned, sliced, and/or peeled; minced garlic in a jar; and dried onion (instead of chopping fresh).

Nutrient Analysis

If a choice of ingredients is given, the first one is used in the nutrient analysis. Ingredients listed as optional are not included in the nutrient analysis. Figures have been rounded. If the value is less than 0.5, it is rounded down to 0. If the figure is 0.5 or more, it is rounded up to 1. The following abbreviations are used in the nutrient listings: g = grams, mg = milligrams. For a list of other measurements, conversions, and abbreviations used in this book, please refer to page 76.

Microwave

Cooking time depends on the microwave wattage, the amount of food being cooked, and the temperature of the food when you start cooking. Only use cookware that is labeled safe for microwave oven use. I prefer to use glass and ceramic containers and avoid use of plastics.

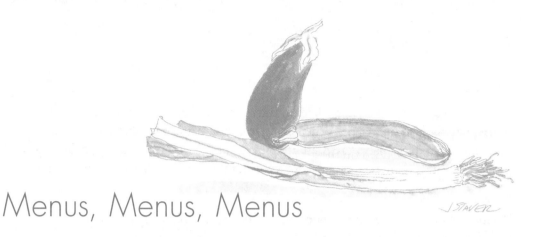

Menus, Menus, Menus

10 Weeks of Dinner Menus—with Grocery Lists

Tips for using

The menus are really quite simple, each one consisting of a protein, a starch (grain, pasta, or starchy vegetable), and a nonstarchy vegetable. Depending on your family's needs, you may also want to add an additional vegetable or another starch, such as a whole-grain roll. Fresh fruit is also a good addition, as desserts are not included. A piece of fresh fruit may be just what you need to satisfy your sweet tooth. Although milk is not listed, it would be a good addition to any meal.

Most of the menu items are recipes from this cookbook. Check the recipes for the yield, and adjust to meet your family's needs. You may want to double a recipe or cut it in half. When serving, adjust portion sizes to meet your individual needs.

Be sure to add to the grocery list the items that you will need for breakfast, lunch, and snacks. Refer to pages 33–34 for ideas that will add variety to breakfast and lunch.

Side dishes

The side dishes that are marked with an asterisk (*) are not in this cookbook. Most are vegetables that can easily be cooked in your microwave (my preference) or steamed. Consult your microwave cookbook for directions. Buy fresh vegetables for the best taste.

These side dishes are on the grocery list with a note to add the amount you need for your family for one meal. You may want to change the side dish and substitute a seasonal food, a family favorite, or a leftover. This is also a good opportunity to take advantage of foods on sale.

Amounts on grocery lists
Amounts listed on the grocery lists are the amounts needed for the recipe and are not always rounded up to full containers or sizes. This way you can check what you have on hand and avoid unnecessary purchases.

Seasonings and staples
Amounts are not included on the grocery list for most seasonings and staples.

Leftovers
Take advantage of leftovers, and serve within a couple of days or freeze for another time. Also freeze in individual portions for lunch. A real timesaving tip is to cook once and serve twice. So consider doubling a recipe..

Abbreviations used on the grocery lists
tsp = teaspoon
Tbsp = tablespoon
oz = ounce
lb = pound

Dinner Menus—Week 1

Ginger Beef • page 249
4 servings
fresh cauliflower* (microwave or steam)
whole-grain roll*

Chicken Parmesan • page 217
6 servings
tossed salad*

Seafood Medley • page 236
4 servings
quick-cooking brown rice*

Taco Salad • page 150
5 servings

Roast Chicken and Vegetables • page 214
4 servings

Week 1—Grocery List

Canned Vegetables, Sauces, & Soups
(To lower sodium, choose no-added-salt or reduced-sodium products.)
chicken broth, fat free (16 oz)
kidney beans (15 oz)
spaghetti sauce (less than 4 g fat
   per 4 oz) 8 oz

Pasta & Rice
fettuccini noodles (8 oz)
quick-cooking brown rice*

Breads & Cereals
whole-grain rolls*

Fresh Produce
green onions (6–8)
onions (1 1/2 medium)
ginger (1 root)
celery (4 stalks)
carrots (2 medium)
red bell pepper (1 1/2 medium)
green bell pepper (1 medium)
snow pea pods, 3 cups (6 oz)
lettuce, 1/2 head (10 oz)
tomatoes (3 medium)
potatoes (4 small)
cauliflower*
salad fixings*

Buy the amount for one meal or substitute a similar food.

Dairy & Cheese

sharp cheddar cheese, reduced fat, grated,
1 cup (4 oz)
mozzarella cheese, reduced fat, grated,
1/2 cup (2 oz)
Parmesan cheese, grated (optional)

Meat, Poultry, & Seafood

beef top sirloin (1 lb)
lean ground beef or ground turkey,
7% fat (1/2 lb)
whole fryer chicken (4–5 lb)
chicken breasts, boneless, skinless (1 lb)
seafood: firm fish (cod, halibut) or scallops,
and/or shelled and deveined shrimp (1 lb)

Seasonings

ground ginger
chili powder
garlic powder
salt (optional)
ground black pepper

Staples

nonstick cooking spray
lite soy sauce
granulated sugar or artificial sweetener
cornstarch
salad dressing, low fat/fat free of your
choice*

Miscellaneous

sherry, white wine or fat-free broth (1 Tbsp)
Thousand Island or ranch-style
dressing (3/4 cup)
tortilla chips, baked (3 oz)

Breakfast foods:

_____

_____

_____

_____

_____

Lunch foods:

_____

_____

_____

_____

_____

Snack foods:

_____

_____

_____

_____

_____

Dinner Menus—Week 2

Curried Sole • page 225
4 servings

**Baked Sweet Potatoes
or Yams** • page 158
4 servings

fresh cooked spinach*
(microwave or steam)

Patio Chicken and Rice • page 213
5 servings

Spicy Pork Burritos • page 255
5 servings

Waldorf Salad • page 140
6 servings

Venus de Milo Soup • page 112
7 servings

whole-grain roll*

Chicken Dijon Fettuccini • page 218
5 servings

tossed salad*

Week 2—Grocery List

Canned Vegetables, Sauces, & Soups
(To lower sodium, choose no-added-salt or reduced-sodium products.)
chicken broth, fat free (16 oz)
beef broth, fat free (40 oz)
mushrooms, sliced (13 oz)
pimento (2 oz)
stewed tomatoes (14.5 oz)
tomato sauce (8 oz)

Pasta & Rice
quick-cooking brown rice (1 1/2 cups)
orzo or quick-cooking barley (3/4 cup)
egg noodles, "no yolk" type (8 oz)

Breads & Cereals
whole-wheat tortillas, 5 (8-inch)
whole-grain rolls*

Fresh Produce
apples (2 medium)
yams or sweet potatoes (2 medium)
carrots, 4 inch (10 small)
green bell pepper (1 medium)
red bell pepper (2 medium)
tomato (1 small)
celery (2 stalks)
onions (1 large & 1 small)
salad fixings*
spinach*

Dairy & Cheese
milk, fat free (3/4 cup)
yogurt, fat free plain (1/4 cup)
cheddar cheese, reduced fat, grated,
   1/2 cup (2 oz)
Parmesan cheese, grated (1 Tbsp)

---

*Buy the amount for one meal or substitute a similar food.

Meat, Poultry, & Seafood
chicken breasts, boneless, skinless (1 lb)
chicken (skinless) thighs, legs and breasts
    (8–10 parts)
pork tenderloin, boneless (1/2 lb)
lean ground beef or ground turkey,
    7% fat (1 lb)
fillets of sole (1 lb)

Seasonings
paprika
dried basil
dried cilantro
dried minced onion
dried parsley
ground cumin
curry powder
salt (optional)
ground black pepper

Staples
nonstick cooking spray
cornstarch
fresh or jar of chopped/minced garlic
lemon juice
light mayonnaise (1/2 cup)
Dijon mustard
salad dressing, low fat/fat free of your
    choice*

Miscellaneous
raisins (1/4 cup)

Frozen Foods
mixed vegetables (16 oz)

Breakfast foods:
_____

_____

_____

_____

_____

Lunch foods:
_____

_____

_____

_____

_____

Snack foods:
_____

_____

_____

_____

_____

Dinner Menus—Week 3

Swiss Steak with Rice • page 251
4 servings

Chicken Cordon Bleu • page 216
4 servings

Creamy Mashed Potatoes • page 160
4 servings

fresh cooked Brussels sprouts*
   (microwave or steam)

Oriental Pork and Noodles • page 254
4 servings

Stuffed Fish Fillets • page 231
4 servings

Cheese Sauce • page 78
1 cup

fresh asparagus* (microwave or steam)

Chicken Chili • page 117
5 servings

raw vegetable slices*

Week 3—Grocery List

Canned Vegetables, Sauces, & Soups
(To lower sodium, choose no-added-salt or reduced-sodium products.)

beef broth, fat free (14 oz)
chicken broth, fat free (22 oz)
tomatoes, diced (29 oz)
water chestnuts, sliced (8 oz)
kidney beans (30 oz)
green chiles, diced (4 oz)

Pasta & Rice
quick-cooking brown rice (1 cup)
coil vermicelli fine noodles (3 oz)

Breads & Cereals
cornflake crumbs (1/4 cup)
unseasoned stuffing mix, cubes
   (3 oz/3 cups)

Fresh Produce
onion (4 medium)
green bell pepper (1 1/2 medium)
red bell pepper (1 1/2 medium)
carrots (3 medium)
potatoes (3 medium)
broccoli, pieces (1 cup)
celery (1 stalk)
asparagus*
Brussels sprouts*
raw vegetable slices*

Dairy & Cheese
milk, fat free (1 1/2 cups)
sour cream, fat free (1/4 cup)
sharp cheddar cheese, reduced fat (2 oz)
Swiss cheese, fat free or reduced fat (2 oz)

Buy the amount for one meal or substitute a similar food.

Meat, Poultry, & Seafood

beef top sirloin (1 lb)
chicken breasts, boneless, skinless (1 1/2 lb)
pork tenderloin, boneless (1 lb)
fish fillets, such as snapper or sole (1 lb)
ham, low fat, 4 slices (1/2 oz each)

Seasonings

dried basil
dried cilantro
dried oregano
dried parsley
dried sage
dried thyme
ground cumin
ground ginger
chili powder
garlic powder
salt (optional)
ground black pepper

Staples

nonstick cooking spray
fresh or jar of chopped/minced garlic
cornstarch
lite soy sauce
unbleached flour

Breakfast foods:

_____

_____

_____

_____

_____

Lunch foods:

_____

_____

_____

_____

_____

Snack foods:

_____

_____

_____

_____

_____

Dinner Menus—Week 4

Beef Stroganoff • page 250
4 servings

fettuccini noodles*
fresh cooked green beans*

Tuna Patties (double recipe) • page 243
4 servings

on whole-wheat hamburger buns
with lettuce and tomato slice*
Cucumbers with Dill Yogurt • page 122
4 servings

Garden Minestrone • page 111
6 servings

whole-grain crackers*

Barbecued Fish Oriental • page 224
4 servings

Grilled Eggplant • page 128
4 servings

baked potato*

**Black Bean and Chicken
Casserole • page 209**
5 servings

Citrus Salad • page 136
5 servings

Week 4—Grocery List

Canned Vegetables, Sauces, Soups, & Fish
*(To lower sodium, choose no-added-salt or
reduced-sodium products.)*
beef broth, fat free (56 oz)
chicken broth, fat free (10 oz)
diced tomatoes (14.5 oz)
green beans (14.5 oz)
black beans (15 oz)
green chiles, diced (4 oz)
tuna packed in water (12 oz)

Pasta & Rice
elbow macaroni (1 cup)
quick-cooking brown rice (1 cup)
fettuccini noodles*

Breads, Cereals, & Crackers
whole-wheat hamburger buns (4)

Fresh Produce
grapefruit (1)
orange (1)
cucumber (1 medium)
cabbage, 1/2 small head (5 oz)
carrots (2 medium)
zucchini (1 small)
eggplant (1 lb)
mushrooms, sliced (1 1/2 cups)
salad greens, 1 1/2 quarts (10–12 oz)
red onion (1 small)
green beans*
baking potatoes*
lettuce and tomato slices*

Dairy & Cheese
sour cream, fat free (1/2 cup)
yogurt, fat free, plain (2 Tbsp)
Parmesan cheese, grated (1 Tbsp)
cheddar cheese, reduced fat, grated,
    1/2 cup (2 oz)

Buy the amount for one meal or substitute a similar food.

Meat, Poultry, & Seafood
beef top sirloin (1 lb)
lean ground beef or ground turkey,
   7% fat (1 lb)
fish fillets (1 lb)
chicken breasts, boneless, skinless (1 lb)

Seasonings
dried basil
dried dill weed
dried chopped/minced onion
dried oregano
dried parsley
onion powder
ground cumin
ground ginger
garlic powder
chili powder
cayenne pepper
salt (optional)
ground black pepper

Staples
nonstick cooking spray
lime juice
lemon juice
light mayonnaise
pickle relish
fresh or jar of chopped/minced garlic
Tabasco sauce
lite soy sauce
ketchup
honey or artificial sweetener
cider vinegar
canola oil
olive oil
unbleached flour

Miscellaneous
orange juice (1/4 cup)
saltines, unsalted top (6 individual)
whole-grain crackers*

Breakfast foods:

_____

_____

_____

_____

_____

Lunch foods:

_____

_____

_____

_____

_____

Snack foods:

_____

_____

_____

_____

_____

Dinner Menus—Week 5

Unstuffed Cabbage Casserole • page 270
4 servings

Chicken Caesar Salad • page 151
4 servings

whole-wheat focaccia bread*

Green Chili Pork Stew • page 115
5 servings

Creamy Seafood Fettuccini • page 235
4 servings

fresh cooked broccoli*
   (microwave or steam)

Spanish Chicken • page 220
4 servings

Spicy Spanish Rice • page 168
5 servings

Week 5—Grocery List

Canned Vegetables, Sauces, & Soups
(To lower sodium, choose no-added-salt or reduced-sodium products.)

chicken broth, fat free (8 oz)
tomato soup, low fat, condensed (10.75 oz)
diced tomatoes (14.5 oz)
salsa, thick and chunky (1/3 cup)
green chiles, diced (11 oz)

Pasta & Rice
quick-cooking brown rice (2 1/2 cups)
egg noodles, "no yolk" type (4 oz)

Breads & Cereals
whole-wheat focaccia bread*

Fresh Produce
onion (1 medium)
red onion (1 small)
green onions (3)
celery (1 stalk)
carrots (2 medium)
potatoes (2 medium)
Romaine lettuce, 1 1/2 quarts (12 oz)
cabbage, 1 small head (1 1/2 lb)
tomato (1 medium)
bell pepper (1 medium)
broccoli*

Dairy & Cheese
milk, fat free (1 1/2 cups)
Parmesan cheese (1/3 cup grated)

Buy the amount for one meal or substitute a similar food.

Meat, Poultry, & Seafood

pork tenderloin, boneless (1 lb)
lean ground beef or ground turkey,
   7% fat (1 lb)
chicken breasts, boneless, skinless (2 lb)
seafood: firm fish (cod, halibut) or scallops,
   and/or shelled and deveined shrimp (1 lb)

Seasonings

dried parsley
dried thyme
ground cumin
ground nutmeg
cayenne pepper
garlic powder
salt (optional)
ground black pepper

Staples

nonstick cooking spray
fresh or jar of chopped/minced garlic
cornstarch
unbleached flour

Miscellaneous

Italian or Caesar dressing, fat free or
   reduced fat (1/4 cup)
sherry, white wine or fat-free chicken
   broth (3 Tbsp)

Breakfast foods:

_____

_____

_____

_____

_____

Lunch foods:

_____

_____

_____

_____

_____

Snack foods:

_____

_____

_____

_____

_____

_____

Dinner Menus—Week 6

Oven Beef Stew • page 113
8 servings

orange slices*

Oriental Seafood • page 239
4 servings

Creamy Chicken Dijon • page 219
4 servings

mashed potatoes*
fresh asparagus* (microwave or steam)

Cornbread Casserole • page 265
6 servings

sliced cucumbers*

Hawaiian Chicken Salad • page 153
4 servings

on lettuce leaves*
fresh fruit slices*

Week 6—Grocery List

Canned Fruits & Juices
pineapple tidbits, in juice (16 oz)

Canned Vegetables, Sauces, & Soups
(To lower sodium, choose no-added-salt or reduced-sodium products.)

tomato juice (1 1/2 cups)
water chestnuts, sliced (16 oz)
chicken broth, fat free (2 cups)
beef broth, fat free (1 cup)

Pasta & Rice
coil vermicelli noodles (3 oz)
quick-cooking brown rice (1 1/2 cups)

Fresh Produce
orange slices*
fresh fruit*
onion (3 medium)
celery (3 stalks)
potatoes (2 medium plus enough for
    mashing for one side dish)
carrots (3 medium)
red bell pepper (2 medium)
broccoli (1 cup pieces)
cucumber*
fresh asparagus*
lettuce leaves*

Dairy & Cheese
egg substitute (1/4 cup, equal to 1 egg)
milk, fat free (3/4 cup)
yogurt, fat free plain (2 Tbsp)

Buy the amount for one meal or substitute a similar food.

Meat, Poultry, & Seafood
round steak (2 lbs)
lean ground beef or ground turkey,
    7% fat (1 lb)
seafood: firm fish (cod, halibut) or scallops,
    and/or shelled and deveined shrimp (1 lb)
chicken breasts, boneless, skinless (2 lb)

Seasonings
bay leaves
chili powder
curry powder
dried oregano
dried parsley
garlic powder
ground black pepper
ground ginger
salt (optional)

Staples
soy sauce
cornstarch
yellow cornmeal
light mayonnaise
Dijon mustard
honey or artificial sweetener
lemon juice
unbleached flour
granulated sugar
baking powder
canola oil

Frozen Foods
mixed vegetables (2 cups)

Miscellaneous
tapioca (2 Tbsp)

Breakfast foods:

_____

_____

_____

_____

_____

Lunch foods:

_____

_____

_____

_____

_____

Snack foods:

_____

_____

_____

_____

_____

Dinner Menus—Week 7

Italian Curry Pasta • page 192
4 servings

Mandarin Cottage Salad • page 139
6 servings

Baked Fish and Rice with
Dill Cheese Sauce • page 233
4 servings
fresh Brussels sprouts*
   (microwave or steam)

Taco Salad • page 150
5 servings

Chicken Medley • page 205
4 servings
whole-wheat roll*

Cheese and Chile
Quesadillas • page 173
4 servings

Black Bean Soup • page 109
4 servings

Week 7—Grocery List

Canned Fruits & Juices
mandarin oranges, in juice (11 oz)
pineapple, crushed, in juice (8 oz)

Canned Vegetables, Sauces, & Soups
chicken bouillon, instant (1 tsp)
chicken broth, fat free (2 cups)
beef broth, fat free (1 1/2 cups)
green chiles, diced (4 oz)
black beans (30 oz)
kidney beans (15 oz)
salsa, thick and chunky (1/2 cup)

Pasta & Rice
angel hair pasta (6 oz)
quick-cooking brown rice (1 cup)

Breads & Cereals
whole-wheat tortillas, 4 (8-inch)
whole-wheat rolls*

Fresh Produce
onions (3 medium)
tomatoes (5 medium)
snow pea pods (3 cups)
celery (4 stalks)
red bell pepper (1 large)
lettuce (1/2 head)
green onions (2)
tomatoes (3 medium)
Brussels sprouts*

Dairy & Cheese
Parmesan cheese, grated (2 Tbsp)
cottage cheese, low fat, small curd (2 cups)
sharp cheddar cheese, reduced fat, grated,
   1 1/2 cup (6 oz)
mozzarella cheese, reduced fat, grated,
   1/2 cup (2 oz)

Buy the amount for one meal or substitute a similar food.

yogurt, fat free, vanilla (8 oz)
milk, fat free (1 1/2 cups)

Meat, Poultry, & Seafood
chicken breasts, boneless, skinless (1 lb)
fish fillets, such as cod or sole (1 lb)
lean ground beef or ground turkey,
   7% fat (1/2 lb)

Seasonings
chili powder
dried cilantro
dried dill weed
dried oregano
dried parsley
garlic powder
ground black pepper
ground cumin
ground ginger
Italian seasoning
onion powder
paprika
salt (optional)

Staples
fresh or jar of chopped/minced garlic
unbleached flour
lite soy sauce
cornstarch

Miscellaneous
orange-flavored gelatin, sugar free
   (2 pkgs, 0.3 oz each)
Thousand Island or ranch-style dressing,
   fat free (3/4 cup)
tortilla chips, baked (3 oz)

Frozen
whipped topping, fat free (1 cup)

Breakfast foods:

_____

_____

_____

_____

_____

Lunch foods:

_____

_____

_____

_____

_____

Snack foods:

_____

_____

_____

_____

_____

Dinner Menus—Week 8

Pork with Apples and Grapes • page 256
5 servings
baked sweet potato or yam*
fresh cooked green beans*

Eggplant Parmesan • page 190
4 servings

Bread Sticks • page 99
12 servings

Seafood Dijon Fettuccini • page 240
5 servings
fresh cooked spinach*
  (microwave or steam)

Chicken and Stuffing Casserole • page 211
6 servings
fresh cooked broccoli*
  (microwave or steam)
whole-berry cranberry sauce*

Creamy Cabbage Soup • page 110
5 servings
rye bread*
sliced fruit*

Week 8—Grocery List

Canned Fruits & Juices
apple cider, unsweetened (1/2 cup)
cranberry sauce, whole berry*

Canned Vegetables, Sauces, & Soups
(To lower sodium, choose no-added-salt or reduced-sodium products.)
spaghetti sauce, less than 4 g fat per 4 oz
  (2 1/2 cups)

Pasta & Rice
egg noodles, "no yolk" type (8 oz)

Breads & Cereals
unseasoned stuffing mix, cubes
  (6 cups/6 oz)
rye bread*

Fresh Produce
apples (2 small)
sliced fruit*
grapes, red seedless (2 cups)
eggplant (1 medium)
red bell pepper (1 large)
cabbage (1 small head)
celery (2 stalks)
onions (2 medium)
green beans*
sweet potato or yam*
fresh spinach*
fresh broccoli*

Dairy & Cheese
mozzarella cheese, reduced fat,
  grated (4 oz)
milk, fat free (3/4 cup)
egg substitute (1/4 cup, equal to 1 egg)

*Buy the amount for one meal or substitute a similar food.

Meat, Poultry, & Seafood
pork tenderloin (1 lb)
seafood: firm fish (cod, halibut) or scallops,
    and/or shelled and deveined shrimp (1 lb)
chicken breasts, boneless, skinless (1 lb)
turkey smoked sausage, reduced fat,
    Polish kielbasa type (8 oz)

Seasonings
dried marjoram
dried parsley
dried sage
dried thyme
ground allspice
ground black pepper
ground cinnamon
salt (optional)

Staples
brown sugar or artificial sweetener
cornstarch
light mayonnaise
Dijon mustard
fresh or jar of chopped/minced garlic
unbleached flour

Frozen
whole-wheat bread dough (1 lb)

Breakfast foods:
_____
_____
_____
_____
_____

Lunch foods:
_____
_____
_____
_____

Snack foods:
_____
_____
_____
_____
_____

Dinner Menus—Week 9

Aloha Chicken • page 221
4 servings

acorn or butternut squash*
fresh cooked asparagus*
  (microwave or steam)

Sour Cream Enchiladas • page 268
8 servings

Citrus Salad • page 136
5 servings

Parmesan Fish Fillets • page 230
4 servings

Oven-Fried Parmesan Potatoes • page 161
5 servings

tossed salad*

Beef Hungarian Goulash (v) • page 204
4 servings

Chicken Chop Suey • page 201
4 servings

quick-cooking brown rice*

Week 9—Grocery List

Canned Fruits & Juices
pineapple slices, in juice (8 oz)

Canned Vegetables, Sauces, & Soups
(To lower sodium, choose no-added-salt or reduced-sodium products.)
chicken or beef broth, fat free (1 1/2 cups)
chicken broth, fat free (1 cup)
green chiles, diced (7 oz)
tomatoes, diced (14.5 oz)
tomato sauce (8 oz)
bean sprouts (16 oz or 1 1/2 cups fresh)

Pasta & Rice
ziti pasta (4 1/2 oz)
quick-cooking brown rice*

Breads & Cereals
whole-wheat tortillas, 8 (8-inch)
bread crumbs, fine (1/4 cup)

Fresh Produce
lemon (1)
grapefruit (1)
orange (1)
green bell pepper (1 large)
greens (1 1/2 quarts)
red onion (1 small)
onions (1 large plus 1 medium)
potatoes (4 medium)
celery (3 stalks)
fresh asparagus*
acorn or butternut squash*
tossed salad*

---

*(v) = variation   *Buy the amount for one meal or substitute a similar food.*

Dairy & Cheese
milk, fat free (1 cup)
sour cream, fat free (1 cup)
Parmesan cheese, grated (1/3 cup)
egg substitute (1/4 cup, equal to 1 egg)

Meat, Poultry, & Seafood
chicken breasts, boneless, skinless (2 lb)
white fish fillets, such as sole, cod,
   snapper (1 lb)
lean ground beef or ground turkey,
   7% fat (1 lb)
top sirloin (1 lb)

Seasonings
chili powder
dried basil
dried parsley
dried thyme
garlic powder
ground black pepper
ground cumin
ground ginger
onion powder
paprika
salt (optional)

Staples
fresh or jar of chopped/minced garlic
cornstarch
Worcestershire sauce
Dijon mustard
lime juice
unbleached flour
cider vinegar
canola oil
molasses
lite soy sauce

Breakfast foods:

_____

_____

_____

_____

_____

Lunch foods:

_____

_____

_____

_____

_____

Snack foods:

_____

_____

_____

_____

_____

Dinner Menus—Week 10

Ramen Chicken • page 206
4 servings

Beef and Cabbage Sandwich
(double recipe) • page 177
4 servings
fresh melon slices*

Tuna Patties (double recipe) • page 243
4 servings

**Creamy Mashed
Potatoes** • page 160
4 servings

**Grilled Vegetable
Medley** • page 129
4 servings

**Skillet Chicken with
Tomatoes** • page 207
4 servings

Italian Baked Fish • page 228
4 servings

**Black Bean Stuffed
Peppers** • page 166
6 servings

Week 10—Grocery List

Canned Vegetables, Sauces, Soups, & Fish
(To lower sodium, choose no-added-salt or reduced-sodium products.)

chicken broth, fat free (4 1/4 cups)
stewed tomatoes (14.5 oz)
black beans (15 oz)
tuna, packed in water (12 oz)

Pasta & Rice
coil vermicelli noodles (4 oz)
quick-cooking brown rice (3/4 cup)

Breads & Cereals
cornflake crumbs (1/4 cup)
pita bread, whole wheat, 2 oz each (4)

Fresh Produce
mushrooms, sliced (1 cup)
carrots (2 medium)
snow pea pods (3 cups)
cabbage (1 small head)
celery (1 stalk)
zucchini (2 small)
red bell pepper (1 medium)
bell peppers, color of your choice
   (3 medium)
potatoes, 6 medium (about 2 lb)
onions (4 medium)
green onions (2)
fresh melon slices*

Dairy & Cheese
milk, fat free (1/4 cup)
sour cream, fat free (1/4 cup)
yogurt, fat free plain (1 cup)
cheddar cheese, reduced fat, grated,
   1/2 cup (2 oz)

Buy the amount for one meal or substitute a similar food.

Meat, Poultry, & Seafood
chicken breasts, boneless, skinless (2 lb)
fish fillets, such as sole, cod, snapper (1 lb)
top sirloin steak (1 lb)

Seasonings
caraway seeds
cayenne pepper
dried oregano
dried parsley
garlic powder
ground black pepper
ground cumin
ground ginger
onion powder
paprika
salt (optional)

Staples
lite soy sauce
cornstarch
Dijon mustard
lemon juice
light mayonnaise
Tabasco sauce
pickle relish
fresh or jar of chopped/minced garlic

Frozen Foods
corn, whole kernel (3/4 cup)

Miscellaneous
saltines, unsalted top (6 crackers)
Italian salad dressing, fat free (1/4 cup)

Breakfast foods:

_____

_____

_____

_____

_____

Lunch foods:

_____

_____

_____

_____

_____

Snack foods:

_____

_____

_____

_____

_____

More Than 100 Easy Menus

When planning meals for the week, choose from these menus below that are listed by category. Serving sizes are listed for each recipe on the recipe page. Adjust the serving size to meet your individual needs. Some recipes are complete meals, in that they have a protein, a vegetable, and a starch. However, you may want to add another item such as a salad, fruit, or whole-grain roll. A glass of fat-free milk is also a good addition to any meal.

Buy fresh vegetables for the side dishes, since these usually taste the best. Serve raw, if appropriate, or simply cook in the microwave or steam.

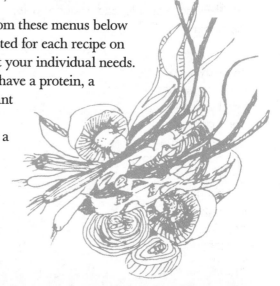

SALADS

Bean and Pasta Salad • page 147
sliced smoked turkey
sliced cucumbers

Turkey Rotini Salad • page 154
sliced fresh fruit

Chicken Caesar Salad • page 151
Focaccia Cheese Bread • page 102

Chicken Rainbow Salad • page 152
on a bed of lettuce
carrot sticks

Hawaiian Chicken Salad • page 153
on lettuce leaves
Grilled Eggplant • page 128

Confetti Shrimp Salad (v) • page 146
sliced tomatoes

Seafood Pasta Salad • page 155
Barbecued Vegetable
   Kabobs • page 126

Tuna Macaroni Salad • page 156
Tomatoes with Yogurt
   Dressing • page 124

Beef, Bean, and Pasta
   Salad • page 149

Taco Salad • page 150

Hot German Potato Salad • page 142
smoked turkey Polish sausage (low-fat)
apple slices

(v) = variation

SANDWICHES

Turkey Reuben Sandwich • page 179
carrot sticks

Chicken Stir-Fry Sandwich • page 178
Spiced Tomato Broth • page 108

Broiled Seafood Muffins • page 175
Summer Coleslaw • page 144

Tuna Patties • page 243
whole-wheat hamburger bun
lettuce and tomato slices
fresh green salad

Tuna Quesadillas • page 174
Waldorf Salad • page 140

Beef and Cabbage
   Sandwich • page 177
fresh melon

Cheese and Chile
   Quesadilla • page 173
tossed salad with garbanzo beans

Black Bean Quesadillas • page 172
sliced raw vegetables

Garden Deli Sandwich • page 180
low-fat cottage cheese

Ricotta Pizza • page 176
tossed salad with kidney beans

Vegetable Stir-Fry
   Sandwich • page 181
Mozzarella and Tomato
   Salad • page 143

SOUPS AND STEWS

Chicken Chili • page 117
raw vegetable sticks

Chicken Pasta Stew • page 118
fresh orange slices

Chicken Soup • page 119
whole-grain roll spread with
light Laughing Cow cheese

Seafood Gumbo • page 116
cornbread

Green Chile Pork Stew • page 115

Oven Beef Stew • page 113
fresh apple slices

Black Bean Soup • page 109
Cheese and Chile
   Quesadillas • page 173

Creamy Cabbage Soup • page 110
rye bread

Garden Minestrone Soup • page 111
whole-grain crackers

Sausage and Lentil Stew • page 114
fresh orange slices

Venus de Milo Soup • page 112
Bread Sticks • page 99

MEATLESS

Broccoli Quiche • page 184
fresh fruit

POULTRY

Chicken and Red Pepper
  Burritos • page 199

Cucumbers with Onions and Sour
  Cream • page 123

Chicken and Stuffing
  Casserole • page 211
fresh cooked Brussels sprouts

Chicken Chop Suey • page 201
noodles or quick-cooking brown rice

Chicken Cordon Bleu • page 216
Creamy Mashed Potatoes • page 160
fresh cooked beets

Chicken Curry • page 202
fresh cooked green beans

Chicken Dijon Fettuccini • page 218
fresh cooked zucchini

Chicken Fricassee • page 203
over mashed potatoes

Chicken Hungarian
  Goulash • page 204

Chicken Medley • page 205
pasta or quick-cooking brown rice

Chicken Noodle Casserole • page 212
fresh cooked broccoli

Chicken Parmesan • page 217
tossed salad

Creamy Chicken Dijon • page 219
baked potato
fresh cooked spinach

Patio Chicken and Rice • page 213
whole cranberry sauce

Ramen Chicken • page 206

Roast Chicken and
  Vegetables • page 214

Skillet Chicken with
  Tomatoes • page 207

Spanish Chicken • page 220
Spanish Rice and Beans • page 167

Szechuan Chicken • page 208
low-fat Ramen noodles

Teriyaki Chicken Breasts • page 215
Grilled Vegetable Medley • page 129
Barbecued Corn on
  the Cob • page 125

Turkey Enchiladas (v) • page 268
Citrus Salad • page 136

Chicken Chili • page 117
raw vegetable sticks

Chicken Pasta Stew • page 118
whole-grain crackers

Chicken Soup • page 119
whole-grain roll spread with
lite Laughing Cow cheese

(v) = variation

Turkey Rotini Salad • page 154
sliced fresh fruit

Chicken Caesar Salad • page 151
Focaccia Cheese Bread • page 102

Chicken Rainbow Salad • page 152
on a bed of lettuce
carrot sticks

Hawaiian Chicken Salad • page 153
on lettuce leaves
Grilled Eggplant • page 128

Turkey Reuben Sandwich • page 179
carrot sticks

Chicken Stir-Fry Sandwich • page 178
Spiced Tomato Broth • page 108

SEAFOOD

Creamy Seafood Fettuccini • page 235
tossed salad

Baked Fish and Rice with Dill Cheese
   Sauce • page 233
fresh cooked broccoli

Barbecued Fish Oriental • page 224
Barbecued Potatoes • page 159
Grilled Eggplant • page 128

Curried Sole • page 225
Zucchini Garden Casserole • page 169

Dijon Fillets • page 226
baked potato
fresh cooked Brussels sprouts

Italian Baked Fish • page 228
Harvest Vegetable Stir-Fry • page 132
whole-grain roll

Mushroom-Topped Fillets • page 229
Baked Sweet Potatoes or
   Yams • page 158
tossed salad

Oriental Seafood • page 239

Creamy Curried Seafood • page 234
pasta or quick-cooking brown rice
raw or fresh cooked carrots

Parmesan Fish Fillets • page 230
Oven-Fried Parmesan
   Potatoes • page 161
fresh cooked beets

Pasta with Clam Sauce • page 241
tossed salad

Seafood Dijon Fettuccini • page 240
fresh cooked spinach

Seafood Medley • page 236
pasta or quick-cooking brown rice

Seafood Pasta • page 237
Cucumbers with Dill Yogurt • page 122

Steamed Clams • page 242
Focaccia Cheese Bread • page 102
tossed salad

Stuffed Fish Fillets • page 231
Cheese Sauce • page 78
fresh cooked green beans

Szechuan Seafood • page 238
low-fat Ramen noodles

Tuna Noodle Casserole • page 244
sliced tomatoes

Fish Poached in Milk • page 227
Black Bean Stuffed Peppers • page 166

Zucchini Fish Bake • page 232
pasta of your choice

Shrimp Burritos • page 245
fresh fruit slices

Tuna Patties • page 243
Creamy Mashed Potatoes • page 160
fresh cooked Brussels sprouts

Confetti Shrimp Salad (v) • page 146
sliced tomatoes

Seafood Pasta Salad • page 155
Barbecued Vegetable
  Kabobs • page 126

Tuna Macaroni Salad • page 156
Tomatoes with Yogurt
  Dressing • page 124

Broiled Seafood Muffins • page 175
Summer Coleslaw • page 144

Tuna Patties • page 243
whole-wheat hamburger bun
lettuce and tomato slices
fresh green salad

Tuna Quesadillas • page 174
Waldorf Salad • page 140

Seafood Gumbo • page 116
cornbread

BEEF AND PORK

Baked Stuffed Pork
  Tenderloin • page 253
fresh cooked asparagus

Beef Hungarian
  Goulash (v) • page 204

Swiss Steak with Rice • page 251

Szechuan Beef • page 252
pasta or brown rice

Beef Stroganoff • page 250
pasta of your choice
tossed salad

Beef Teriyaki • page 248
Barbecued Corn on the
  Cob • page 125
Barbecued Zucchini • page 127

Ginger Beef • page 249
fresh cooked broccoli
quick-cooking brown rice

(v) = variation

GROUND MEAT AND SAUSAGE

Menu Ideas for Breakfast and Lunch

The ideas listed below will add variety to your breakfast and lunch. Page numbers are listed for recipes in this book. For additional suggestions for breakfast and lunch that don't require a recipe, refer to my previous title, *Quick & Healthy Recipes and Ideas, 3rd Edition*.

Breakfast

For a balanced breakfast, include:

- Fruit or fruit juice. Fruit has more fiber than juice, so it is the better choice.
- Whole-grain breads and/or cereals. Look on the label for "whole wheat" or "whole grain." Best choices have 3 or more grams of fiber per serving and less than 3 grams of fat for 100 calories.
- Fat-free or low-fat dairy products and/or other low-fat protein-rich foods from the meat group. Protein is important at breakfast because it has "staying power," which means it stays with you longer than most other foods, so you feel full for a longer period of time—hopefully until lunch.

Use some of the following recipes and suggestions to add variety to your breakfast.

Spanish Quiche, page 186

Vegetarian Sausage Quiche, page 185

Sausage and Egg Casserole, page 262

Ricotta Pizza, page 176

Pear Custard (v), page 276

Peach Custard, page 276

Baked Grape-Nuts Pudding, page 274

Raisin Bread Pudding, page 275

Applesauce Bread Pudding (v), page 275

Carrot Muffins, page 95

Apple Cider Pancakes, page 92

Banana Bread, page 93

Date Nut Bread, page 96

Pineapple Bread, page 97

Pumpkin Bread, page 98

Buttermilk Bran Breakfast Bars, page 94

Fat-free yogurt with sliced fruit

Fat-free yogurt with sliced fruit, sprinkled with Grape Nuts cereal or any ready-to-eat whole-grain cereal

Peanut butter spread on whole-grain toast

Assorted whole-grain breads such as whole-wheat bagels, whole-wheat English muffins, whole-wheat toast

Assorted whole-grain cereals (hot and cold)

Low-fat cottage cheese or low-fat ricotta cheese with fruit

French toast (made with whole-grain bread)

Hot cereal topped with fat-free yogurt, nuts, and fruit

Scrambled eggs or omelets

(v) = variation

Lunch

For a balanced lunch, include:

- Starchy food such as whole-grain breads, tortillas, crackers, bagels, pasta, or starchy vegetables such as potatoes
- Fruits and/or nonstarchy vegetables such as salad, tomatoes, carrots, etc.
- Low-fat protein-rich foods from the meat group (includes beans) and/or fat-free or low-fat dairy products

Use some of the following recipes and suggestions to add variety to your lunch.

Beef and Cabbage Sandwich, page 177

Garden Deli Sandwich, page 180

Tuna Quesadillas, page 174

Black Bean Quesadillas, page 172

Tuna Patties, page 243 (serve on a whole-wheat bun)

Vegetable Stir-Fry Sandwich, page 181

Turkey Reuben Sandwich, page 179

Spiced Tomato Broth, page 108 (serve with a sandwich)

Ricotta Pizza, page 176

Chicken Soup, page 119

Tortilla Soup, page 107 (serve with a soft taco)

Tuna Macaroni Salad, page 156

Confetti Shrimp Salad (v), page 146

Chicken Caesar Salad, page 151

Seafood Pasta Salad, page 155

Tossed salad with garbanzo or kidney beans

Sandwiches made with low-fat meats and low-fat cheeses

Turkey sandwich with sliced tomato and green chiles

Fruit plate with sliced low-fat cheese

Tuna salad on a whole-wheat bagel

Sliced low-fat meats and cheese with sliced vegetables

Melon with low-fat cottage cheese

Leftovers, especially soups and casseroles

(v) = variation

 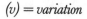

Changing Recipes . . .
to Reduce Fat, Sugar, and Calories

You can make your favorite recipes healthier with just a few changes.

High Calorie/High Fat	Better Choice
Frying	Try broiling, poaching, baking, or frying in a nonstick pan. A nonstick spray also works well. Use fat-free broth as a substitute for oil when cooking chopped onions and other vegetables.
High-fat breadings	Use cornflake crumbs.
Tuna packed in oil	Try water-packed tuna.
Chicken cooked with skin	Remove skin from chicken either before or after cooking.
Red meats	Trim all fat before cooking. Serve only three times a week and limit portions to 3–4 ounces.
Ground meats	Choose ground beef and ground turkey with 7% fat or less.
Cheddar and high-fat cheese	Use low-fat, light, or reduced-fat cheese.
Sour cream	Use plain fat-free yogurt or fat-free sour cream.
Whole milk	Choose a lower-fat milk. Compare calories for 1 cup: Fat-free milk: 85 calories; 1% milk: 100 calories; 2% milk: 120 calories; whole milk: 155 calories.
Cream cheese for dips	Use low-fat or fat–free cream cheese. Also try low-fat cottage cheese or low-fat ricotta cheese. Blend with fat-free milk and add seasonings.
Canned fruit in heavy syrup	Use fresh fruit or fruit in natural juices without added sugar.
Fried tortillas	Heat in oven, wrapped in foil; or heat in microwave between two microwave-safe plates.
Soups	Refrigerate. The fat will rise to the top and harden. Remove the fat before serving.
Gelatins	Use sugar-free gelatin.
Butter and margarine	Try butter-flavored sprinkles on vegetables.
Mayonnaise	Use low-fat, light, or reduced-fat mayonnaise.
Salad dressing	Use fat-free, light, or reduced-fat salad dressings.
Refried beans	Buy fat free.

Tips for Eating Out

You don't have to eat every meal at home to be successful at limiting fat and/or calories. Here are some ideas and food choices to keep in mind when you eat out.

Plan Ahead

Save up calories by eating lighter earlier in the week and/or having smaller portions for breakfast and lunch. However, don't skip a meal.

Ask Questions

When scanning a menu, focus on the better choices. Don't be afraid to ask for special preparations. Communication is the key.

First Course

Go with fresh fruit, vegetable juice, or consommé. Avoid cream soups.

Side Salads

Leafy salads are always a good choice. The thinner salad dressings, such as Italian, are the best choice, since you can use less. Ask for your salad dressing on the side or use a lemon wedge, or simply carry your own. A salad that comes coated with dressing adds as many as 500 calories. Be sure to avoid croutons, sunflower seeds, cheese, and cold salads such as potato and macaroni.

Salad Bars

Fill up on lettuce, tomatoes, mushrooms, green peppers, onions, cucumbers, carrots, cauliflower, broccoli, celery, and radishes. Limit ham, croutons, cheese, nuts, seeds, and high-fat dressings. Use a low-calorie dressing or lemon wedge. If the salad bar is all you will be eating, choose to add lean meat slices and kidney and garbanzo beans for protein. Also refer to the Salad Bar Guide on page 38.

Order à la Carte

Don't feel like you have to order a complete meal. Choose two items from the appetizer list, such as steamed clams and a salad, and ask for a roll. Order just what you want. By ordering less food, you will eat less!

Avoid Fried Foods

Calories more than double in foods that are deep-fried. Cut down on fat in fried foods by removing the outer crust before eating.

Pizza

If you can limit yourself to one or two pieces, a good choice is cheese with veggies such as green peppers, onions, mushrooms, and tomatoes. Add a salad.

Entrées

Choose an entrée that is broiled, grilled, poached, or roasted. Always ask if you are not sure. Go with lean meats and fish. Steer clear of fried foods, rich sauces, and gravy. These are all sources of unwanted calories and fat.

Extras

- Ask whether vegetables are prepared with added butter or sauce. If they are, ask that yours be prepared without.

- Baked potatoes are great, but limit or omit sour cream, butter, and bacon bits.

- You don't have to eat something just because it comes with your order. You can always remove the batter from fish or the skin from chicken.

Eat Half

Split a sandwich or meal with a friend or take half home.

Avoid Mayonnaise

Order a plain hamburger or sandwich with tomato, lettuce, and pickle and skip the mayonnaise. One tablespoon of mayonnaise has 100 calories.

Limit Desserts

Desserts can be a potential disaster zone. Limit your portion or try fresh fruit. Share a dessert with a friend.

Limit or Avoid Alcoholic Beverages

Alcohol increases your appetite and decreases your willpower. Try a non-calorie club soda with a twist of lemon or lime. A 6-ounce wine spritzer has about 65 calories. To make a make a wine spritzer, mix 3 ounces of dry wine with 3 ounces of diet soda such as ginger ale.

Avoid High-Calorie Beverages

Regular soft drinks add 150 calories and milkshakes easily add 400 calories. Order low-calorie beverages such as fat-free milk, non-calorie soft drinks, and water.

Drop Out of the Clean Plate Club

You don't have to finish everything on your plate! Moderation is the key to success.

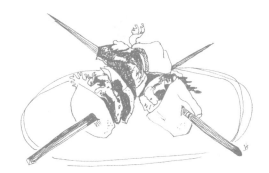

Salad Bar Guide

Choose carefully to limit unwanted calories and fat. Use the information below to make better choices.

Start with: 1 cup combined = fewer than 20 calories (Exchange = "free")	Add liberally: 1 cup combined = 25 calories (Exchange = 1 nonstarchy vegetable)	Enjoy but don't overdo:

Lettuce
Spinach
Green onion
Mushrooms
Zucchini
Celery
Cucumber
Hot pepper
Radishes
Dill pickles (high sodium)
	Green peppers
	Cauliflower
	Purple onion
	Carrots
	Broccoli
	Tomato
		Fruit
		Melon, 1 cup
		    60 calories
		    (1 fruit exchange)
		Other fruit, 1/2 cup
		    60 calories
		    (1 fruit exchange)

Add sparingly:
About 1/2 cup, level

Item	Calories	Exchange
Cottage cheese	90	2 lean meat
Macaroni salad	295	2 carbohydrate, 3 fat
Potato salad	165–250	1 1/2–2 carbohydrate, 1–2 fat
Pasta salad	295	2 carbohydrate, 3 fat
Bean salad	170	1 carbohydrate, 1 lean meat, 1 fat
Coleslaw	150	1 carbohydrate, 1 1/2 fat
Pickled beets	75	1 carbohydrate

Add sparingly:

Item	Amount	Calories
Peas	1 tablespoon	10
Soy bacon bits	1 tablespoon	20
Chow Mein noodles	1 tablespoon	30
Croutons	2 tablespoons	20
Egg	1 tablespoon	15
Cheddar cheese	1 tablespoon	30
Turkey ham	1 tablespoon	25
Olives	1 tablespoon	15
Raisins	1 tablespoon	30
Parmesan cheese	1 tablespoon	25
Sunflower seeds	1 tablespoon	50
Crackers	1 package (2 crackers)	26 (1/2 starch)

Carefully measure:
About 1 level tablespoon

Item	Calories	Exchange
Ranch	80	2 fat
Thousand Island	60	1 1/2 fat
Bleu cheese	80	2 fat
Dijon	90	2 fat
Italian	40	1 fat
French	75	2 fat
Reduced-fat French	20	1/2 fat
Reduced-fat Thousand Island	30	1 fat
Reduced-fat Italian	30	1 fat
Reduced-fat ranch	40	1 fat

Helpful Party Tips

If you are struggling with weight control, use some of these tips to help you to be successful at a party.

Plan Ahead

Think about how much you will eat before you arrive at the party. You will not feel deprived if you limit your calories earlier in the week and that day, so you will be able to eat more while at the party. However, do not skip meals and limit yourself so much that you arrive starving.

Position Yourself

Stand by the fireplace and not by the food. It's not an issue of motivation. It's your plan to limit temptation.

Socialize

Put the emphasis on people instead of food.

Appetizers

Munch on raw vegetables instead of nuts, chips, or other high-calorie foods. If you are tempted to indulge in other appetizers, choose one that is your favorite, and eat only half as much as you normally would.

Hold Something

Busy hands can't hold food in them, so keep your hands busy by holding something. It could be anything from a napkin to a glass of water.

Portion Sizes

Be food-wise at dinner. Take smaller portions of higher-calorie foods and larger portions of vegetables and green salads.

Alcohol

If you enjoy a cocktail, limit yourself to one. Choose wine mixed with diet soda pop or alcohol mixed with water or diet soda pop to limit extra calories. Club soda with a twist of lemon is really your best choice. And remember, alcohol stimulates your appetite!

Eat Slowly

Put your fork down between mouthfuls. Stop eating when you feel satisfied, not when you feel stuffed.

Dessert

Just have a small serving. And remember, you don't have to eat it all. You can always say, "Your wonderful dinner filled me up."

Buffets

If dinner is a buffet, look over the entire array of food before deciding. Allow yourself one serving of everything if it can fit on your plate without being heaped. Have smaller portions of higher-calorie foods. No seconds!

Don't Get Discouraged

Keep a proper perspective. If you eat more than what you had intended, don't overwhelm yourself with guilt. Think of it as a learning experience. Ask yourself, "What did I learn to help me do better next time?" Pick yourself up and get back in control right away!

Lastly, have fun and enjoy the party.

Trim Calories from Your Holiday Dinner

Holidays are a wonderful time for family and sharing. However, if these times cause unwanted weight gain, consider the following tips to help you.

Serve Lighter Appetizers

Many appetizers are high in fat and fill you up before you even start the meal. Change your favorite recipes by substituting lower-fat ingredients such as low-fat or fat-free yogurt and sour cream. Use fruits and vegetables with dips and spreads, instead of chips or crackers.

> For variety and color, arrange a combination of any of the following: cucumber, kohlrabi, and zucchini slices; sliced green, red, and yellow bell peppers; celery and carrot sticks; broccoli and cauliflower florets; and cherry tomatoes. Serve with a low-fat ranch dressing for dipping.

Avoid Self-Basting Turkeys

A self-basting turkey, which has been injected with added fat or oil, could have as many as 2,400 additional calories, depending on the size of the bird.

Avoid the Skin

The skin keeps the turkey moist while it's roasting, but it's loaded with fat. An ounce of roasted turkey skin is about 100 calories, mostly from fat. So forgo eating the skin, and save the calories for dessert.

Limit Stuffing or Change Your Recipe

Traditional stuffing is high in fat because of all the butter or margarine. Limit yourself to one small serving, and you will save yourself a lot of calories. Better yet, make a fat-free dressing by substituting broth for the margarine or butter in your recipe. It tastes just as good! You can also add more celery and onion to your recipe to further reduce calories.

Lighten the Mashed Potatoes

Use fat-free milk or fat-free ranch dressing instead of whole milk or half and half. You can further reduce calories by using butter-flavored sprinkles instead of margarine.

Make Fat-Free Gravy

Pour pan drippings into a glass measuring cup and let set until the fat rises. Every tablespoon of fat skimmed off has 130 calories. Thicken your gravy with cornstarch instead of flour and save more calories.

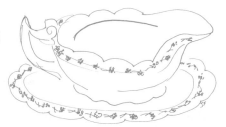

Fat-Free Gravy

1 cup cold broth, fat removed
2 tablespoons flour (or 1 tablespoon cornstarch)
seasonings to taste

Pour 1/4 cup broth in a covered container. Add flour and shake well to avoid lumps. In a small saucepan, combine remainder of broth with the flour mixture. Heat on medium, stirring constantly with a wire whisk, until bubbly and thickened. Season to taste.

Avoid Extras

Pass up the candied or creamed vegetables, or at least limit your portion. Choose a vegetable without a rich sauce. For a buttery flavor, use a small amount of butter-flavored sprinkles. It has only 4 calories per 1/2 teaspoon.

Approach Salads with Caution

Salads are great as long as they are not made with regular cream cheese, sour cream, mayonnaise, or cream. Your best choices would be a fresh green salad or fruit salad. Add your own dressing lightly.

Don't Make Dessert a Danger Zone

Plan on making a dessert that is not high in fat. There are several recipes in this book that you and your family will enjoy. And remember, no matter what you have for dessert, moderation is important.

Pumpkin Pie Tip

For something more traditional, try lightening your favorite pumpkin pie recipe by substituting evaporated skim milk and egg substitute. Make it with the traditional single crust, or lower the calories even more by eliminating the crust. If you are making a crustless pie, be sure to spray the pie pan with nonstick cooking spray before pouring in the filling. This will prevent sticking and make it easier to serve. Top each slice with a dollop of fat-free whipped topping before serving.

Think Smaller

If tradition dictates that you have some dishes that are high calorie or high fat, you can still cut your calories in half by having a smaller portion. Also, avoid the temptation to double the portion of dishes that are lower in calories.

Enjoy!

Eat slowly and put your fork down while chewing. Really take the time to enjoy the food you are eating. Enjoy each mouthful!

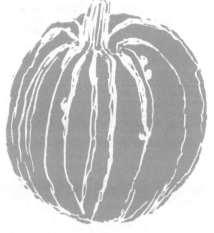

Determining Your Healthy Weight and Calorie Needs

By following the steps below, you can determine your desirable weight and approximate calorie needs. In the next section, you can then determine the upper limit of fat recommended for your calorie level.

Step 1: Determine a Healthy Weight

Using the Adult BMI* Chart below, determine a healthy weight for your height. If you already know what weight is good for you, skip this step and go to Step 2.

*BMI (body mass index) is determined by a formula that uses both an individual's height and weight.

Adult BMI Chart

Locate your height in the left-most column and read across the row for that height to your present weight. Follow the column of the weight, up to the top row that lists the BMI.

	Normal						Overweight					Obese									
BMI	19	20	21	22	23	24	25	26	27	28	29	30	31	32	33	34	35	36	37	38	39
Height										Body Weight (pounds)											
4'10"	91	96	100	105	110	115	119	124	129	134	138	143	148	153	158	162	167	172	177	181	186
4'11"	94	99	104	109	114	119	124	128	133	138	143	148	153	158	163	168	173	178	183	188	193
5'0"	97	102	107	112	118	123	128	133	138	143	148	153	158	163	168	174	179	184	189	194	199
5'1"	100	106	111	116	122	127	132	137	143	148	153	158	164	169	174	180	185	190	195	201	206
5'2"	104	109	115	120	126	131	136	142	147	153	158	164	169	175	180	186	191	196	202	207	213
5'3"	107	113	118	124	130	135	141	146	152	158	163	169	175	180	186	191	197	203	208	214	220
5'4"	110	116	122	128	134	140	145	151	157	163	169	174	180	186	192	197	204	209	215	221	227
5'5"	114	120	126	132	138	144	150	156	162	168	174	180	186	192	198	204	210	216	222	228	234
5'6"	118	124	130	136	142	148	155	161	167	173	179	186	192	198	204	210	216	223	229	235	241
5'7"	121	127	134	140	146	153	159	166	172	178	185	191	198	204	211	217	223	230	236	242	249
5'8"	125	131	138	144	151	158	164	171	177	184	190	197	203	210	216	223	230	236	243	249	256
5'9"	128	135	142	149	155	162	169	176	182	189	196	203	209	216	223	230	236	243	250	257	263
5'10"	132	139	146	153	160	167	174	181	188	195	202	209	216	222	229	236	243	250	257	264	271
5'11"	136	143	150	157	165	172	179	186	193	200	208	215	222	229	236	243	250	257	265	272	279
6'0"	140	147	154	162	169	177	184	191	199	206	213	221	228	235	242	250	258	265	272	279	287
6'1"	144	151	159	166	174	182	189	197	204	212	219	227	235	242	250	257	265	272	280	288	295
6'2"	148	155	163	171	179	186	194	202	210	218	225	233	241	249	256	264	272	280	287	295	303
6'3"	152	160	168	176	184	192	200	208	216	224	232	240	248	256	264	272	279	287	295	303	311
6'4"	156	164	172	180	189	197	205	213	221	230	238	246	254	263	271	279	287	295	304	312	320

Adapted from Clinical Guidelines on the Identification, Evaluation, and Treatment of Overweight and Obesity in Adults: The Evidence Report. National Institutes of Health. 1998.

Interpreting Your BMI

Healthy weight	Overweight	Obese
BMI of 18.5–24.9	BMI of 25–29.9	BMI of 30 and above

Limitations of the BMI: 1. BMI does not differentiate between muscle and fat; 2. Very muscular individuals may appear to be overweight, when they are not; 3. Fat may be underestimated for individuals who have lost muscle mass.

Healthy Weight Range

If your BMI is in the healthy weight range, use your present weight in Step 3.

Example: Sue is 5'6" tall and weighs 136 pounds. She determines that her BMI is 22 and in the healthy weight range. She will use her present weight in Step 3.

Overweight or Obese Range

If you are in the overweight or obese range, go back to the chart and again locate your height in the left-most column and read across the row for your height to the weight that is at the upper end of the healthy weight range. Use that weight for Step 3. This may not be your most desirable weight but it is a good starting goal.

Example: Sue is 5'6" tall and weighs 167 pounds. She determines that her BMI of 27 is in the overweight range. She will use 148 pounds in Step 3.

Step 2: Choose Your Activity Level

From the table below, choose the activity level that best describes your lifestyle. Next to your activity level is the approximate number of calories a person typically burns per pound of body weight. Extremely active people will require additional calories.

Calorie Needs

Activity Level	Calories per Pound
Very Active*	17
Moderately Active**	15
Inactive***	13

*Very active: Daily routine includes both sitting and walking and light housework/yard work, plus aerobic exercise equivalent to brisk walking more than 3 miles every day.

**Moderately active: Daily routine includes both sitting and walking and light housework/yard work, plus aerobic exercise equivalent to a 1.5- to 3-mile brisk walk every day.

***Inactive: Daily routine includes some walking but mostly sitting; no additional exercise.

Example: Sue is a businesswoman who walks briskly 2–3 miles everyday. In addition, she does light housework on weekends and some yard work.

Below is Sue's activity level and calories needed for her activity.
Activity level: ___Moderately Active___ Calories per pound: _15_

List your activity level and calories needed for your activity.
Activity Level: _____ Calories per pound: ____

Step 3: Estimate Your Calorie Needs
Complete the formula below with the information you have so far.

Example:
Sue's calorie needs:

136 pounds	Healthy body weight (Step 1)
× 15	Calories per pound for activity level (Step 2)
2,040	Calories needed per day

Your calorie needs:

_____ pounds	Healthy body weight (Step 1)
×_____	Calories per pound for activity level (Step 2)
	Calories needed per day

Note: This is only an estimate. Your actual calorie needs will vary depending on a number of factors such as your age, body build, metabolism, and additional amounts of exercise.

Adjusting Calories for Weight Loss or Weight Gain

• To lose weight:

Subtract 500 calories per day from your calorie needs figured above.

Note: The figure 500 is flexible. Even a reduction of 100 calories a day will lead toward success. So, do what will work for you. Keep in mind that a moderate reduction in calories combined with increased exercise is usually the best way to lose weight.

It is recommended that women eat at least 1,200 calories per day and that men eat at least 1,500 calories per day.

• To gain weight:

Add 500 calories per day to your calorie needs figured above.

Note: The figure 500 is flexible. Even an increase of 100 calories a day will lead toward success. So, do what will work for you.

Example:

Adjusting Sue's calories:

For weight loss: 2,040 calories (Step 3) − (minus) 500 calories = 1,540 calories needed per day

For weight gain: 2,040 calories (Step 3) + (plus) 500 calories = 2,540 calories needed per day

Adjusting your calories:

For weight loss: _____calories (Step 3) − (minus) 500 calories =_____ calories needed per day

For weight gain: _____calories (Step 3) + (plus) 500 calories = _____ calories needed per day

---

Consult a registered dietitian for help with determining your ideal weight and an individualized plan to help you reach your goal.

Determining Your Daily Limit of Fat

The information below will help you to determine the amount of fat recommended for your calorie level.

The general recommendation for how much total fat is acceptable is between 20 and 35% of your total calories for the day. For those needing to lose weight, it is recommended not to exceed 30%.

Saturated fat, which is part of the total fat, should be limited to less than 7–10% of your total calories. The American Heart Association recommends limiting saturated fats to less than 7% of total calories.

Note: *Total fat includes saturated fat as well as monounsaturated, polyunsaturated, and trans fats.*

Your physician should advise you as to what is an appropriate total fat and saturated fat intake for your individual needs.

Although a low-fat diet is healthy, some individuals take low-fat eating to the extreme and try to eat a no-fat diet. This is not desirable, since it can interfere with the optimum balance of nutrients needed for good health.

Monounsaturated and polyunsaturated fats are your best choices. These are known to lower blood cholesterol levels when part of a low-fat diet.

- Monounsaturated fats: Main sources are canola oil, olive oil, peanut oil, avocado, olives, almonds, cashews, peanuts, pecans, and sesame seeds.
- Polyunsaturated fats: Main sources are corn oil, safflower oil, soybean oil, sunflower oil, and sunflower seeds.
- Omega-3 fats are a type of polyunsaturated fat. Main sources are salmon, walnuts, flaxseed, and soybean oil.

Both saturated fats and trans fats are known to increase blood levels of cholesterol.

- Saturated fats should be limited. Main sources of saturated fat are animal sources, palm oil, coconut oil, and hydrogenated fats.
- Trans fats should be avoided. You can do this by knowing what to look for on food labels. Main sources of trans fats are commercially prepared items such as chips, cookies, crackers, and muffins that contain the words "hydrogenated" or "partially hydrogenated" in the list of ingredients. Fortunately, many food companies are eliminating trans fats in their processed foods.

The table below lists daily calories, grams of total fat representing 20–30% of daily calories, and grams of saturated fat representing 7% of daily calories. *Note: Although saturated fat is listed separately, it is also included in the total fat.*

Recommended Daily Limit of Grams of Fat		
Calories per day	Grams of total fat (20–30% of total calories)	Grams of saturated fat (7% of total calories)
1,200	27–40	9
1,400	31–47	11
1,600	36–53	12
1,800	40–60	14
2,000	44–67	16
2,200	49–73	17
2,400	53–80	19
2,600	58–87	20
2,800	62–93	22
3,000	67–100	23

Using the above table:
- Find the calorie level in the first column that is closest to what you have determined in Step 3 beginning on page 47.
- In the second column, find the amount of total fat listed for your calorie level.
- Next, go to the third column and find the amount of saturated fat listed for your calorie level.

Example:
For Sue: 2,040 Calories   44–67 grams of total fat (20–30% of total calories)
                           16 grams of saturated fat (7% of total calories)

Yours: _____ Calories   _____ grams of total fat (20–30% of total calories)
                         _____ grams of saturated fat (7% of total calories)

Once you know the grams of fat that are acceptable for you, compare this figure with what you are actually eating. Refer to the next section "Monitoring Fat."

Monitoring Fat

There are two convenient sources for finding the grams of fat in what you eat: *1)* food labels found on almost every food product and *2)* books and tables that list grams of fat in foods. The sections "Grams of Fat in Common Foods" and "Looking at Food Labels for Fat" will help you find the amount of fat in foods you typically eat.

After reviewing these two sections, go on to the "Sample Food Record" on page 62. Use this as a guide to complete your own food record using the form on page 63.

Using the Food Record

Make additional copies of this form. You will need one for each day of recordkeeping. To complete your Food Record, list the foods you eat in a day and the grams of total fat in each food. Add up your fat grams for the day and compare it to the recommended amount you listed on page 50. You can do the same for saturated fat. However, you will be pleased to know that, in most cases, when you restrict your total fat, your saturated fat intake also decreases.

Remember that your weekdays and weekends may be very different. To get a true picture, you really need to look at both.

It's natural that the amount of fat you eat will vary from day to day. However, your ultimate goal should be to keep the average amount of fat that you eat over a one-week period of time within the range recommended for you.

Reducing Your Fat Intake

If you are eating too much fat, refer to the section "Grams of Fat in Common Foods" on page 53 and find lower-fat alternatives. Also check out the section "Trimming Fat from Your Diet" on page 60.

As you continue to look at labels, you will find more foods that are low in fat. Keep in mind that most fruits and vegetables are virtually fat free and are good low-calorie, high-fiber choices. Your higher-fat foods tend to be processed foods such as fried foods, frozen breaded products, cookies, pastries, chips, and fast foods.

By keeping fat at a healthy level, you are not only protecting your cardiovascular system, but you are also keeping calories in check.

Fat and Weight Loss

Many people have lost considerable weight simply by reducing the amount of fat they eat, and it's no secret why this works. Fat is more calorically dense than carbohydrate or protein. Fat has 9 calories per gram, whereas carbohydrate and protein have only 4 calories per gram.

Cutting back on fat and increasing fruits and vegetables is a good way to lose weight. This has worked for many. However, a low-fat diet is not always the total solution. Too many calories, regardless of the source, cause weight gain.

Get Help

As you make changes, seek help from a registered dietitian who has the background to help you make changes that are realistic for you.

Grams of Fat in Common Foods

Below is a listing of common foods and the approximate grams of total fat and saturated fat for the serving size listed. Note that grams of saturated fat are also included in the total fat grams. Use this chart as a guide, but be sure to read food labels, since the amount of fat will vary with different brands.

Breads and Grains

FOOD	AMOUNT	TOTAL FAT GRAMS	SATURATED FAT GRAMS
Bagel (2 oz)	1	1	*
Bread, whole wheat, white	1 slice	1	*
English muffin, whole wheat	1	1	*
Croissant (1.5 oz)	1	12	7
Noodles/pasta	1/2 cup	*	*
Oatmeal, cooked	1 cup	2	*
Pancake (4-inch diameter)	3	3	1
Rice, brown	1/2 cup	1	*
Tortilla, flour (7–8-inch)	1	1–3	0–1
Tortilla, corn (6-inch)	1	1	*
Total cereal	3/4 cup	1	*
Wheaties	1 cup	1	*

Fruits and Vegetables

FOOD	AMOUNT	TOTAL FAT GRAMS	SATURATED FAT GRAMS
Avocado	1/8	4	*
Baked potato	1 medium	*	*
French fries, deep fried	10	9	3
French fries, frozen–oven baked	10	4	1
Fruit: fresh, canned, or juice	1/2 cup	*	*
Vegetables: fresh, canned, or frozen	1/2 cup	*	*

Beans (Legumes) and Nuts

FOOD	AMOUNT	TOTAL FAT GRAMS	SATURATED FAT GRAMS
Baked beans, vegetarian	1 cup	1	*
Garbanzo beans	1/2 cup	1	*
Kidney beans	1/2 cup	*	*
Pinto beans	1/2 cup	*	*
Refried beans, fat free	1/2 cup	*	*
Nuts:			
Almonds (22)	1 oz	15	1
Cashews (18)	1 oz	13	2
Hazelnuts/filberts (20)	1 oz	17	1
Peanuts (28)	1 oz	14	2

*Indicates less than 1/2 gram of fat.

 FAT GRAMS IN COMMON FOODS |

FOOD	AMOUNT	TOTAL FAT GRAMS	SATURATED FAT GRAMS
Pecans (20 halves)	1 oz	21	2
Walnuts, English (14 halves)	1 oz	19	2
Peanut butter, regular	1 Tbsp	8	2
Peanut butter, reduced fat	1 Tbsp	6	1

Dairy

FOOD	AMOUNT	TOTAL FAT GRAMS	SATURATED FAT GRAMS
Cheeses:			
Cottage cheese, regular	1/2 cup	5	3
Cottage cheese, 2%	1/2 cup	2	1
Cottage cheese, 1%	1/2 cup	1	1
Cream cheese, regular	2 Tbsp	10	6
Cream cheese, light	2 Tbsp	5	3
Cream cheese, fat free	2 Tbsp	*	*
Cheddar, Swiss, American	1 oz	9	6
Mozzarella, part skim	1 oz	5	3

FOOD	AMOUNT	TOTAL FAT GRAMS	SATURATED FAT GRAMS
Parmesan cheese	2 Tbsp	3	2
Reduced-fat cheddar, Swiss, etc.	1 oz	6	3
Milk:			
Whole	1 cup	8	5
2%	1 cup	5	3
1%	1 cup	3	2
Fat free	1 cup	*	*
Sour cream:			
Regular	1 Tbsp	3	2
Reduced fat	1 Tbsp	2	1
Fat free	1 Tbsp	*	*
Yogurt:			
Low fat	1 cup	4	2
Fat free	1 cup	*	*

Eggs

FOOD	AMOUNT	TOTAL FAT GRAMS	SATURATED FAT GRAMS
Egg, large	1	5	2
Egg substitute, fat free	1/4 cup	*	*

Meat, Poultry, and Seafood

FOOD	AMOUNT	TOTAL FAT GRAMS	SATURATED FAT GRAMS
Beef:			
Ground, 7% fat	3 oz	8	3
Ground, 10% fat	3 oz	10	4

Indicates less than 1/2 gram of fat.

FOOD	AMOUNT	TOTAL FAT GRAMS	SATURATED FAT GRAMS
Ground, 15% fat	3 oz	13	5
Ground, 20% fat	3 oz	15	6
Ground, 25% fat	3 oz	16	6
Prime rib	3 oz	30	12
Top sirloin, select, lean only	3 oz	5	2
Top sirloin, choice, lean only	3 oz	7	3
Elk steak	3 oz	3	1
Venison steak	3 oz	3	1
Lamb, roast-lean only	3 oz	7	3
Pork:			
Bacon, crisp	2 slices	6	1
Top loin (meat and fat)	3 oz	10	4
Top loin (lean only)	3 oz	6	2
Ham, regular	3 oz	11	4
Ham, 95% fat free	3 oz	1	*
Tenderloin (lean only)	3 oz	4	1
Poultry:			
Chicken white meat	3 oz	3	1
Chicken dark meat	3 oz	8	2

FOOD	AMOUNT	TOTAL FAT GRAMS	SATURATED FAT GRAMS
Fried chicken	3 oz	18	5
Ground turkey, 7% fat	3 oz	7	2
Turkey, white meat	3 oz	3	1
Turkey, dark meat	3 oz	9	3
Sausage and sandwich meats:			
Bologna, beef and pork	1 oz	8	3
Bologna, turkey	1 oz	4	1
Hot dogs, regular	1	13	5
Hot dogs, fat free	1	*	*
Salami, beef and pork	1 oz	5	2
Salami, turkey	1 oz	4	1
Sandwich meat, 95% fat free	1 oz	1	*
Sausage links, beef or pork	2.4 oz	21	8
Smoked sausage/kielbasa:			
Regular	2 oz	10	4
Reduced-fat turkey	2 oz	5	2
Seafood:			
Crab, shrimp, scallops (no shell)	3 oz	1	*

*Indicates less than 1/2 gram of fat.

 FAT GRAMS IN COMMON FOODS | 55

FOOD	AMOUNT	TOTAL FAT GRAMS	SATURATED FAT GRAMS
Clams (no shell)	3 oz	2	*
Fried fish, shrimp, scallops	3 oz	15	4
Oysters (no shell)	3 oz	2	*
Salmon, Chinook	3 oz	11	3
Tuna fish, water pack	3 oz	2	*
White fillets, snapper and sole	3 oz	2	*

Fats and Oils

FOOD	AMOUNT	TOTAL FAT GRAMS	SATURATED FAT GRAMS
Butter	1 tsp	4	2
Margarine	1 tsp	4	1
Margarine, light	1 tsp	2	1
Mayonnaise, regular	1 Tbsp	11	2
Mayonnaise, light	1 Tbsp	5	1
Mayonnaise, fat free	1 Tbsp	*	*
Oil, canola	1 Tbsp	14	1
Oil, olive	1 Tbsp	14	2
Salad dressings:			
Bleu cheese, regular	1 Tbsp	8	2
Bleu cheese, reduced fat	1 Tbsp	2	*

FOOD	AMOUNT	TOTAL FAT GRAMS	SATURATED FAT GRAMS
Italian, regular	1 Tbsp	7	1
Italian, fat free	1 Tbsp	*	*
Ranch, regular	1 Tbsp	8	1
Ranch, reduced fat	1 Tbsp	4	*

Snacks and Desserts

FOOD	AMOUNT	TOTAL FAT GRAMS	SATURATED FAT GRAMS
Apple pie	1/8 pie	14	5
Chips, baked tortilla	1 oz	1	*
Chips (fried): potato, corn, tortilla	1 oz	10	3
Chips (light): potato	1 oz	6	1
Cake, angel food	1 oz	*	*
Cake doughnut	1	11	2
Glazed doughnut	1	14	4
Chocolate chip cookie (2 1/4-inch)	1	2	1
Fig bar	1	1	*
Gingersnaps, graham crackers, vanilla wafers	2	1	*
Ice cream, regular	1/2 cup	8	5
Ice cream, light	1/2 cup	4	2
Sherbet	1/2 cup	2	1

Indicates less than 1/2 gram of fat.

56 | **QUICK & HEALTHY II**

FOOD	AMOUNT	TOTAL FAT GRAMS	SATURATED FAT GRAMS
Sorbet/ Italian ice	1/2 cup	*	*
Popsicle	1	*	*
Popcorn, popped, no butter added:			
Air popped	3 1/2 cups	1	*
Popped with oil	2 1/2 cups	8	1
Microwave, butter	3 cups	8	2
Microwave, light butter	3 cups	3	*
Pretzels	1 oz	1	*
Rice cakes	1	*	*

Fast Food**

FOOD	AMOUNT	TOTAL FAT GRAMS	SATURATED FAT GRAMS
Hamburgers:			
Cheeseburger, regular	1	14	6
Hamburger, regular	1	12	4
McDonald's Quarter Pounder	1	19	7
McDonald's Big Mac	1	29	10
Burger King Whopper	1	40	11
Chicken:			
Burger King TenderGrill chicken sandwich with mayo	1	19	4

FOOD	AMOUNT	TOTAL FAT GRAMS	SATURATED FAT GRAMS
Fried chicken, drumstick and thigh	2 pieces	27	7
McDonald's Crispy Chicken Sandwich	1	20	4
McDonald's Grilled Chicken Sandwich	1	10	2
McDonald's Chicken McNuggets	6	17	3
Taco Bell Spicy Chicken Soft Taco	1	6	2
Taco Bell Chicken Fiesta Taco Salad	1	38	8
McDonald's Egg McMuffin	1	12	5
McDonald's Sausage McMuffin with Egg	1	27	10
Fish sandwich (fried)	1	23	5
French fries, regular	1 order	25	5
Pizza, pepperoni	1 slice	7	2
Taco Bell Taco Supreme	1	13	6

*Indicates less than 1/2 gram of fat.   **Ordering without mayonnaise or high-fat sauces will significantly lower the fat.*

Looking at Food Labels for Fat

The food label lists the total fat for one serving as well as other information.

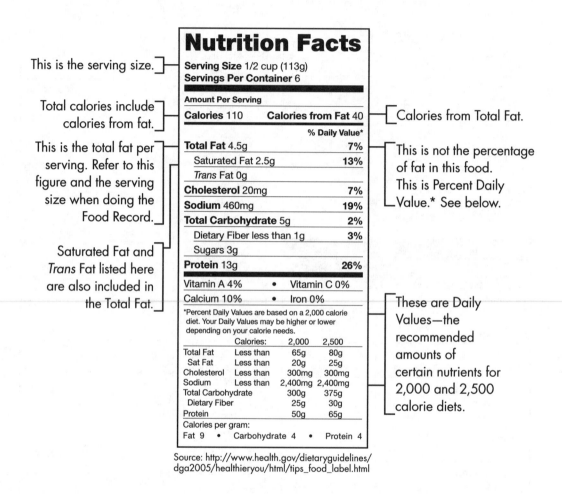

This is the serving size.

Total calories include calories from fat.

This is the total fat per serving. Refer to this figure and the serving size when doing the Food Record.

Saturated Fat and *Trans* Fat listed here are also included in the Total Fat.

Nutrition Facts

Serving Size 1/2 cup (113g)
Servings Per Container 6

Amount Per Serving

Calories 110	**Calories from Fat** 40

	% Daily Value*
Total Fat 4.5g	**7%**
Saturated Fat 2.5g	**13%**
Trans Fat 0g	
Cholesterol 20mg	**7%**
Sodium 460mg	**19%**
Total Carbohydrate 5g	**2%**
Dietary Fiber less than 1g	**3%**
Sugars 3g	
Protein 13g	**26%**

Vitamin A 4%	•	Vitamin C 0%
Calcium 10%	•	Iron 0%

*Percent Daily Values are based on a 2,000 calorie diet. Your Daily Values may be higher or lower depending on your calorie needs.

	Calories:	2,000	2,500
Total Fat	Less than	65g	80g
Sat Fat	Less than	20g	25g
Cholesterol	Less than	300mg	300mg
Sodium	Less than	2,400mg	2,400mg
Total Carbohydrate		300g	375g
Dietary Fiber		25g	30g
Protein		50g	65g

Calories per gram:
Fat 9 • Carbohydrate 4 • Protein 4

Calories from Total Fat.

This is not the percentage of fat in this food. This is Percent Daily Value.* See below.

These are Daily Values—the recommended amounts of certain nutrients for 2,000 and 2,500 calorie diets.

Source: http://www.health.gov/dietaryguidelines/ dga2005/healthieryou/html/tips_food_label.html

Serving Size Is Important

To accurately determine the grams of fat for a food, check the serving size to see whether it is the amount you typically eat. It is not unusual for people to eat two or more servings, thinking they are eating only one. This is especially true when the serving size is 1/2 cup. At this point, you may need to get out a measuring cup to be sure.

Example:	1 serving	= 1/2 cup	= 4.5 grams total fat
	2 servings	= 1 cup	= 9 grams total fat

Follow the General Rule

Choose foods with less than 3 grams of total fat for each 100 calories, and that is for total calories not calories from fat. When this is not possible, balance higher-fat foods with low-fat or fat-free foods.

Percent of Fat

The percent of calories from fat in one serving of food is not listed on the label. If you want to calculate this, divide the total calories from fat by the total calories and multiply by 100.

Example: 40 calories from fat ÷ 110 total calories × 100 = 36% of calories from fat

Trimming Fat from Your Diet

You can trim fat from your diet by using these suggestions.

- Choose only lean meats, and trim all visible fat before cooking.

- Remove the skin from chicken and turkey.

- Choose lean beef with 7% fat or less.

- Choose ground turkey with 7% fat or less.

- Look for meat that has little or no marbling of fat.

- Avoid high-fat meats such as bacon, bologna, and salami.

- Avoid foods fried in oil or other fats.

- Use a nonstick cooking spray for frying or a spray pump filled with canola or olive oil.

- Sauté foods in a few tablespoons of broth, fruit juice, or water.

- Bake, broil, simmer, microwave, or barbecue.

- Skim fat from homemade and canned soups. Refrigerate, and the fat will harden and rise to the top for easy removal.

- Limit use of margarine on vegetables; try a dash of butter-flavored sprinkles instead.

- Use a fruit spread or fat-free cream cheese on toast instead of margarine.

- Use lettuce and tomato on sandwiches instead of mayonnaise.

- Avoid high-fat snacks such as potato chips, corn chips, corn curls, pastries, and rich desserts.

- Avoid all foods with trans fats. These are commercially processed foods that have the words "hydrogenated" or "partially hydrogenated" in the list of ingredients.

- Substitute the following reduced-fat or fat-free foods for higher-fat foods.

  Fat-free or 1% milk

  Evaporated fat-free milk

  Fat-free yogurt (plain or flavored)

  Ice milk

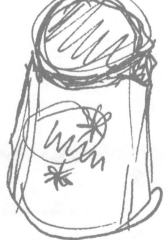

Light or fat-free sour cream

Light or fat-free cream cheese

Reduced-fat or fat-free mayonnaise

Reduced-fat or fat-free salad dressings

Reduced-fat, low-fat, or fat-free cheeses

Reduced-fat margarine

Fat-free tartar sauce

Water-packed tuna

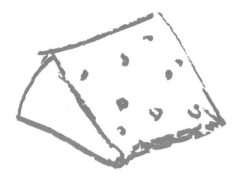

- Substitute low-fat snacks for traditional high-fat snacks.
  (Look for no more than 3 grams of fat for every 100 calories.)

  Pretzels, both hard and soft (salt-free available)

  Light microwave popcorn

  Air-popped popcorn

  Fresh fruit

  Low-fat ice milk

  Low-fat frozen yogurt

  Frozen juice bars

  Rice cakes

  Corn cakes (caramel flavor is great)

  Tomato juice with a twist of lemon (try no-salt-added)

  Raw vegetable sticks with fat-free salad dressing for a dip

  Low-fat crackers and cookies

  Graham crackers, vanilla wafers, gingersnaps, animal crackers, fig bars

  Unsalted-top saltines

  Fat-free hot cocoa

  Sugar-free soda pop with a scoop of low-fat ice milk

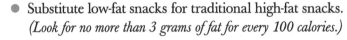

Sample Food Record

Date: _March 6_

In addition to recording foods eaten, include fat used in cooking as well as sandwich spreads, salad dressings, and anything you put on the food.

Food	Amount	Grams of Total Fat
fresh orange juice	1/2 cup	0
oatmeal, cooked	1 cup	2
fat-free milk	1 cup	0
whole-wheat toast	1 slice	1
fruit spread	2 tsp	0
banana	1	0
sandwich		
whole-wheat pita bread	1	1
water-packed tuna	3 oz	2
lettuce and tomato slices	several of each	0
light mayonnaise	3 Tbsp	15
carrot and celery sticks	5 sticks each	0
apple	1	0
Teriyaki Chicken Breasts (page 215)	1 serving	3
baked potato	1	0
sour cream, fat free	2 Tbsp	0
broccoli	1 cup	0
butter-flavored sprinkles	dash	0
tossed salad	1 serving	0
ranch dressing, reduced fat	2 Tbsp	8
garbanzo beans for salad	1/2 cup	1
whole-wheat roll	1	1
margarine	1 tsp	4
fat-free milk	1 cup	0
gingersnaps	8 small	4
light microwave-popped popcorn	6 cups	6
	Total Fat:	48
	Recommended Limit:	44-67
	Over:	0

Food Record

Date:_____

In addition to recording foods eaten, include fat used in cooking as well as sandwich spreads, salad dressings, and anything you put on the food.

Food	Amount	Grams of Total Fat
	Total Fat:	
	Recommended Limit:	
	Over:	

Food Exchanges for Diabetes and Weight Loss

Exchange lists are used in many weight-loss programs and diabetic diets. In forming the exchange lists, foods with similar calories, carbohydrate, protein, and fat are grouped together.

By following a meal pattern based on the exchange lists, one can "exchange" a food in one group for another food in the same group. This method helps to increase variety while at the same time keeping calories and nutrient values fairly consistent.

The basic exchange lists are:

Carbohydrates

Starch–includes breads, cereals, grains, starchy vegetables, and crackers

Fruit

Milk–includes milk and yogurt

Sweets, desserts, and other carbohydrates

Nonstarchy vegetables

Meat and Meat Substitutes (also includes cheese)

Lean

Medium-fat

High-fat

Plant-based proteins

Fats

The Meat and Meat Substitutes list and the Milk list are further divided into groups based on the amount of fat a food contains. The leanest meats and the fat-free/low-fat dairy products are the best choices.

Please be aware that the calories, carbohydrate, protein, and fat used for each exchange list are averages and are not always the exact values for a specific food within the exchange list.

Foods with less than 20 calories and 5 grams or less of carbohydrate per serving are listed as "free" for one serving. If you eat more than one serving, the food is not considered "free" and should be counted as an exchange.

Each recipe in this book has the exchanges listed. The figures used to calculate the exchanges are from *Choose Your Foods: Exchange Lists for Diabetes* by the American Diabetes Association and American Dietetic Association.

Carb Servings

All recipes in this book include Carb Servings, also known as Carb Choices. The general rule is: 15 grams of carbohydrate equals 1 Carb Serving.

Talk to your registered dietitian or diabetes educator about adjusting the carbohydrate if a serving/portion of food has more than 5 grams of fiber.

NOTE: Carb Servings and Exchanges listed for the recipes have been adjusted for fiber. In some recipes, this resulted in no change. If the fiber is more than 5 grams, half of the grams of fiber are subtracted from the total grams of carbohydrate when figuring Exchanges and Carb Servings.

The following chart was used to convert carbohydrate to Carb Servings.

Carbohydrate Grams	Carb Servings
0–5	0
6–10	1/2
11–20	1
21–25	1 1/2
26–35	2
36–40	2 1/2
41–50	3
51–55	3 1/2
56–65	4

J.S.

Recipes Listed by Carbohydrate

The following is a table listing recipes that are grouped by grams of carbohydrate. This can be especially helpful for people with diabetes when planning meals around a specific number of grams of carbohydrate. It is also helpful for people in weight-loss programs who need calories, grams of fat, and dietary fiber for their calculations.

You can adjust your serving size, which will increase or decrease the grams of carbohydrate per serving, to meet your individual needs.

This listing includes calories, fat, carbohydrate, carb servings, and fiber.

Carb servings listed have been adjusted for fiber. In some recipes, this resulted in no change. If the fiber is more than 5 grams, half of the grams of fiber are subtracted from the total grams of carbohydrate when figuring exchanges and carb servings.

Below is the number of recipes listed by grams of carbohydrate in the table that follows:

33 recipes	0–5 grams of carbohydrate
22 recipes	6–10 grams of carbohydrate
39 recipes	11–20 grams of carbohydrate
17 recipes	21–25 grams of carbohydrate
61 recipes	26–35 grams of carbohydrate
21 recipes	36–40 grams of carbohydrate
8 recipes	41–50 grams of carbohydrate

Recipes Listed by Grams of Carbohydrate

One portion of the following recipes has 0–5 grams of carbohydrate and is counted as 0 Carb Servings.

	One Serving	Calories	Total Fat Grams	Carbo-hydrate Grams	Dietary Fiber Grams	Carb Servings
APPETIZERS AND SAUCES						
Pimento and Cheese Spread	1 Tbsp	34	2	1	0	0
Herbed Cream Cheese	2 Tbsp	40	1	1	0	0
Tuna Paté	2 Tbsp	34	0	1	0	0
Dijon Sauce	1 Tbsp	26	2	2	0	0
Veggie Spread	2 Tbsp	28	1	2	0	0
Cream Cheese Spread	2 Tbsp	26	0	2	0	0
Cucumber Spread	2 Tbsp	18	0	2	0	0
Cheese Sauce	2 Tbsp	40	1	3	0	0
Dill Cheese Sauce (v)	2 Tbsp	40	1	3	0	0
Bean and Cheese Dip	2 Tbsp	30	0	4	1	0
Bean and Salsa Dip	2 Tbsp	24	0	4	1	0
Chili Cheese Dip	2 Tbsp	32	0	4	1	0
Layered Black Bean Dip	2 Tbsp	32	1	5	1	0
SOUPS AND STEWS						
Sherried Broth	1 cup	19	0	3	0	0
VEGETABLES						
Barbecued Zucchini	1/4 recipe	12	0	2	1	0
Cucumbers with Dill Yogurt	1/2 cup	35	2	3	1	0
Cucumbers with Onions and Sour Cream	1/2 cup	18	0	4	1	0
Barbecued Vegetable Kabobs	1/4 recipe	23	0	5	1	0
Italian Green Beans	1/2 cup	26	0	5	2	0
Green Bean Sauté	1/2 cup	27	0	5	2	0
SALADS						
Mozzarella and Tomato Salad	1/4 recipe	72	4	5	1	0
POULTRY						
Teriyaki Chicken Breasts	1/4 recipe	132	3	1	0	0
Creamy Chicken Dijon	1/4 recipe	174	7	3	0	0
Spanish Chicken	1/4 recipe	147	3	4	1	0
SEAFOOD						
Dijon Fillets	1/4 recipe	135	4	1	0	0
Fish Poached in Milk	1/4 recipe	118	2	2	0	0

(v) = variation

	One Serving	Calories	Total Fat Grams	Carbo-hydrate Grams	Dietary Fiber Grams	Carb Servings
Barbecued Fish Oriental	1/4 recipe	119	2	2	0	0
Curried Sole	1/4 recipe	147	6	2	0	0
Mushroom-Topped Fillets	1/4 recipe	122	2	3	1	0
Steamed Clams	1/3 recipe	133	2	5	0	0
BEEF AND PORK						
Beef Teriyaki	1/4 recipe	139	5	1	0	0
Ginger Beef	1/2 cup	157	5	5	0	0
DESSERTS						
Popsicles	1	3	0	0	0	0

One portion of the following recipes has 6–10 grams of carbohydrate and is counted as 1/2 Carb Serving.

SOUPS AND STEWS						
Spiced Tomato Broth	1 cup	41	0	7	2	1/2
VEGETABLES						
Grilled Vegetable Medley	1/4 recipe	29	0	6	2	1/2
Harvest Vegetable Stir-Fry	1/2 cup	36	1	6	1	1/2
Tomatoes with Yogurt Dressing	1/2 cup	35	1	6	1	1/2
Grilled Eggplant	1/4 recipe	62	3	7	0	1/2
Ranch-Style Vegetables	1/2 cup	49	0	10	2	1/2
SALADS						
Summer Coleslaw	1/2 cup	43	2	6	1	1/2
Chicken Caesar Salad	1/4 recipe	168	4	6	2	1/2
POULTRY						
Chicken Cordon Bleu	1/4 recipe	186	3	7	0	1/2
Szechuan Chicken	1 1/2 cups	232	9	9	3	1/2
Aloha Chicken	1/4 recipe	172	3	10	0	1/2
SEAFOOD						
Creamy Curried Seafood	1/2 cup	145	2	7	1	1/2
Zucchini Fish Bake	1/4 recipe	157	2	8	2	1/2
Tuna Patties	1 patty	170	6	8	0	1/2
Italian Baked Fish	1/4 recipe	142	2	8	0	1/2
Parmesan Fish Fillets	1/4 recipe	164	4	6	0	1/2
Szechuan Seafood	1 1/2 cups	211	7	9	3	1/2

	One Serving	Calories	Total Fat Grams	Carbo-hydrate Grams	Dietary Fiber Grams	Carb Servings
BEEF AND PORK						
Szechuan Beef	1 cup	199	9	8	2	1/2
Beef Stroganoff	3/4 cup	187	5	9	1	1/2
DESSERTS						
Mandarin Yogurt Delight	1/2 cup	40	0	7	0	1/2
Strawberry Yogurt Mousse	1/2 cup	45	0	9	1	1/2
Peach Popsicles	1	40	0	10	1	1/2

One portion of the following recipes has 11–20 grams of carbohydrates and is counted as 1 Carb Serving.

	One Serving	Calories	Total Fat Grams	Carbo-hydrate Grams	Dietary Fiber Grams	Carb Servings
BREADS						
Focaccia Veggie Bread	1/16 recipe	77	2	13	3	1
Focaccia Cheese Bread	1/16 recipe	87	2	13	3	1
Bread Sticks	1	106	2	18	2	1
SOUPS AND STEWS						
Seafood Gumbo	1 1/2 cups	163	2	14	2	1
Tortilla Soup	1 1/4 cups	79	1	14	1	1
Creamy Cabbage Soup	1 1/2 cups	155	4	15	2	1
Chicken Soup	1 1/2 cups	142	1	18	2	1
SALADS						
Waldorf Salad	1/2 cup	73	3	12	1	1
Fruit Cocktail Salad	1/2 cup	57	0	13	1	1
Citrus Salad	1 1/2 cups	96	3	15	6	1*
Mandarin Cottage Salad	3/4 cup	128	1	15	0	1
Black Bean Salad	1/2 cup	81	0	16	2	1
Broccoli and Raisin Salad	1/2 cup	132	5	18	2	1
Frozen Fruit Salad	1/2 cup	80	0	19	1	1
Seafood Pasta Salad	1 cup	159	4	19	1	1
Tuna Macaroni Salad	1 cup	151	1	20	2	1
Hot German Potato Salad	1/2 cup	100	1	20	2	1
POTATOES, RICE, BEANS, AND PASTA						
Baked Sweet Potatoes or Yams	1/2 potato	60	0	14	2	1
Spanish Rice and Beans	1/2 cup	85	1	16	2	1
Seasoned Black Beans	1/3 cup	103	0	18	3	1

*Carb Servings listed have been adjusted for fiber. In some recipes this resulted in no change. If the fiber is more than 5 grams, half of the grams of fiber are subtracted from the total grams of carbohydrate when figuring Exchanges and Carb Servings.

 CARBOHYDRATE IN RECIPES |

	One Serving	Calories	Total Fat Grams	Carbo-hydrate Grams	Dietary Fiber Grams	Carb Servings
SANDWICHES						
Broiled Seafood Muffins	1 half	136	4	14	2	1
Chicken Stir-Fry Sandwich	1/4 recipe	147	2	15	1	1
Beef and Cabbage Sandwich	1/2 sandwich	180	3	19	1	1
Vegetable Stir-Fry Sandwich	1/2 sandwich	129	1	20	2	1
MEATLESS ENTREES						
Broccoli Quiche	1/8 recipe	134	3	13	1	1
Vegetarian Sausage Quiche	1/8 recipe	157	4	14	1	1
POULTRY						
Chicken Fricassee	1 cup	216	3	14	2	1
Chicken Chop Suey	1 1/4 cups	197	3	15	2	1
Chicken à la King	3/4 cup	214	4	16	2	1
Chicken Medley	1 1/2 cups	207	3	16	3	1
SEAFOOD						
Seafood Medley	1 1/2 cups	186	2	15	2	1
Stuffed Fish Fillets	1/4 recipe	197	2	19	1	1
BEEF AND PORK						
Sweet and Sour Pork	1 cup	212	4	18	2	1
GROUND MEAT AND SAUSAGE						
Sausage and Egg Casserole	1/6 recipe	148	5	11	2	1
DESSERTS						
Pumpkin Cheesecake	1/12 recipe	86	0	12	0	1
Strawberry Delight	3/4 cup	60	0	12	1	1
New York Cheesecake	1/12 recipe	94	0	14	1	1
Chocolate Peanut Butter Frozen Bars	1 bar	122	4	18	0	1
Glazed Fruit Cup	1 cup	80	0	19	2	1
Layered Mousse	3/4 cup	105	0	20	0	1

One portion of the following recipes has 21–25 grams of carbohydrate and is counted as 1 1/2 Carb Servings.

	One Serving	Calories	Total Fat Grams	Carbo-hydrate Grams	Dietary Fiber Grams	Carb Servings
BREADS						
Mexican Cornbread	1/9 recipe	169	6	22	2	1 1/2
SOUPS AND STEWS						
Oven Beef Stew	1 cup	220	4	23	3	1 1/2
Garden Minestrone Soup	1 1/2 cups	245	6	25	5	1 1/2

	One Serving	Calories	Total Fat Grams	Carbo-hydrate Grams	Dietary Fiber Grams	Carb Servings
Chicken Pasta Stew	1 1/2 cups	223	3	25	2	1 1/2
SALADS						
Turkey Rotini Salad	1 cup	169	2	22	2	1 1/2
POTATOES, RICE, BEANS, AND PASTA						
Dijon Fettuccini	1/2 cup	144	4	24	1	1 1/2
Szechuan Pasta	3/4 cup	145	3	23	2	1 1/2
SANDWICHES						
Tuna Quesadillas	1/4 recipe	229	6	24	1	1 1/2
Cheese and Chile Quesadillas	1/4 recipe	173	3	25	1	1 1/2
MEATLESS ENTREES						
Spanish Quiche	1/8 recipe	180	4	21	2	1 1/2
Eggplant Parmesan	1/4 recipe	188	5	24	3	1 1/2
BEEF AND PORK						
Pork with Apples and Grapes	1 cup	195	4	22	2	1 1/2
GROUND MEAT AND SAUSAGE						
Sweet and Sour Beans	1/2 cup	142	2	21	5	1 1/2
DESSERTS						
Applesauce Bread Pudding (v)	1/9 recipe	118	1	23	3	1 1/2
Baked Grape-Nuts Pudding	1/2 cup	126	0	24	1	1 1/2
Chocolate Vanilla Swirl Pie	1/8 recipe	187	7	25	1	1 1/2
Strawberry-Pineapple Shortcake	1/8 recipe	113	0	25	1	1 1/2

One portion of the following recipes has 26–35 grams of carbohydrates and is counted as 2 Carb Servings.

BREADS						
Drop Biscuits	1	165	4	28	1	2
Traditional Biscuits (v)	1	169	4	28	1	2
Apple Cider Pancakes	2	144	1	30	1	2
Date Nut Bread	1/16 recipe	156	2	32	1	2
Biscuit Wedges (v)	1	185	4	32	1	2
Pineapple Bread	1/9 recipe	158	1	33	2	2
Banana Bread	1/9 recipe	166	1	35	3	2
Buttermilk Bran Breakfast Squares	1/9 recipe	169	1	35	5	2

(v) = variation

	One Serving	Calories	Total Fat Grams	Carbo-hydrate Grams	Dietary Fiber Grams	Carb Servings
SOUPS AND STEWS						
Chicken Chili	1 1/4 cups	236	2	33	10	2*
Black Bean Soup	1 1/4 cups	171	1	30	6	2*
Venus de Milo Soup	1 1/2 cups	262	5	33	5	2
VEGETABLES						
Barbecued Corn on the Cob	1 ear	136	1	28	3	2
SALADS						
Hawaiian Chicken Salad	1 1/2 cups	294	9	28	2	2
Confetti Salad	1 cup	132	1	28	2	2
Confetti Shrimp Salad (v)	1/5 recipe	218	2	28	2	2
Vegetable Pasta Salad	1 cup	146	1	30	2	2
Bean and Pasta Salad	1 cup	188	2	33	4	2
Rainbow Vegetable Salad	1/6 recipe	195	3	33	3	2
Chicken Rainbow Salad	1 1/4 cups	297	8	34	3	2
Taco Salad	2 cups	302	9	34	6	2*
POTATOES, RICE, BEANS, AND PASTA						
Black Bean Stuffed Peppers	1/6 recipe	160	3	26	4	2
Spicy Spanish Rice	1 cup	131	1	27	1	2
Creamy Dill Fettuccini	1/2 cup	170	3	27	1	2
Barbecued Potatoes	1/4 recipe	126	0	29	3	2
Oven-Fried Parmesan Potatoes	1/5 recipe	159	3	29	3	2
Zucchini Garden Casserole	1/4 recipe	149	1	30	3	2
Creamy Mashed Potatoes	1/2 cup	136	0	31	3	2
SANDWICHES						
Ricotta Pizza	1/6 recipe	200	4	31	2	2
Garden Deli Sandwich	1 sandwich	221	1	35	4	2
Vegetable Pita Sandwich	1 sandwich	243	6	32	2	2
Turkey Reuben Sandwich	1 sandwich	272	6	28	5	2
MEATLESS ENTREES						
Cheese and Tortilla Lasagna	1/6 recipe	220	4	29	2	2
POULTRY						
Black Bean and Chicken Casserole	1 1/4 cups	252	4	26	4	2
Chicken and Red Pepper Burritos	1/5 recipe	226	5	27	1	2

*Carb Servings listed have been adjusted for fiber. In some recipes this resulted in no change. If the fiber is more than 5 grams, half of the grams of fiber are subtracted from the total grams of carbohydrate when figuring Exchanges and Carb Servings.

(v) = variation

	One Serving	Calories	Total Fat Grams	Carbo-hydrate Grams	Dietary Fiber Grams	Carb Servings
Chicken and Broccoli in Cheese Sauce	1/5 recipe	302	6	27	3	2
Chicken and Stuffing Casserole	1/6 recipe	230	3	27	1	2
Turkey Enchiladas (v)	1/8 recipe	256	6	29	2	2
Skillet Chicken with Tomatoes	1 1/2 cups	255	3	29	4	2
Chicken Parmesan	1/6 recipe	271	4	33	2	2
SEAFOOD						
Baked Fish and Rice/Dill Cheese Sauce	1/4 recipe	301	5	27	1	2
Shrimp Burritos	1/5 recipe	216	4	28	1	2
Tuna Noodle Casserole	3/4 cup	238	4	30	2	2
Oriental Seafood	1 3/4 cups	260	2	31	4	2
Creamy Seafood Fettuccini	1 cup	310	4	32	1	2
BEEF AND PORK						
Spicy Pork Burritos	1/5 recipe	225	5	26	1	2
Oriental Pork and Noodles	1 3/4 cups	285	5	31	3	2
Baked Stuffed Pork Tenderloin	1/4 recipe	317	6	35	1	2
GROUND MEAT AND SAUSAGE						
Italian Baked Ziti	1 cup	231	4	30	2	2
Sour Cream Enchiladas	1/8 recipe	276	8	29	2	2
Pasta Olé	1/4 recipe	287	7	34	2	2
South of the Border Lasagna	1/8 recipe	305	7	35	3	2
Cornbread Casserole	1/6 recipe	319	10	35	4	2
Unstuffed Cabbage Casserole	2 cups	336	10	36	6	2*
DESSERTS						
Raisin Bread Pudding	1/9 recipe	141	1	27	3	2
Chocolate Cream Pie	1/8 recipe	156	3	27	0	2
Pear Custard (v)	1/9 recipe	130	0	28	3	2
Chocolate Peanut Butter Pie (v)	1/8 recipe	206	7	29	1	2
Banana Cream Pie	1/7 recipe	157	3	29	1	2
Peach Custard	1/9 recipe	133	0	29	2	2
Baked Pears with Chocolate Sauce	1 pear	133	1	33	5	2
Apple Crisp Parfait	1/4 recipe	149	1	35	3	2

*Carb Servings listed have been adjusted for fiber. In some recipes this resulted in no change. If the fiber is more than 5 grams, half of the grams of fiber are subtracted from the total grams of carbohydrate when figuring Exchanges and Carb Servings.

(v) = variation

 CARBOHYDRATE IN RECIPES |

One portion of the following recipes has 36–40 grams of carbohydrates and is counted as 2 1/2 Carb Servings.

	One Serving	Calories	Total Fat Grams	Carbo-hydrate Grams	Dietary Fiber Grams	Carb Servings
BREADS						
Carrot Muffins	1	163	1	36	1	2 1/2
Pumpkin Bread	1/9 recipe	187	1	40	3	2 1/2
SOUPS AND STEWS						
Green Chile Pork Stew	1 1/2 cups	269	4	37	4	2 1/2
Sausage and Lentil Stew	1 cup	228	2	40	5	2 1/2
SALADS						
Beef, Bean, and Pasta Salad	1 1/2 cups	294	7	43	6	2 1/2*
SANDWICHES						
Black Bean Quesadillas	1/4 recipe	250	4	38	3	2 1/2
MEATLESS ENTREES						
Rice and Bean Burritos	1/8 recipe	215	2	40	3	2 1/2
POULTRY						
Chicken Noodle Casserole	1 1/2 cups	285	3	37	2	2 1/2
Ramen Chicken	1 3/4 cups	318	4	37	3	2 1/2
Chicken Dijon Fettuccini	1 1/3 cups	316	7	37	2	2 1/2
Chicken Curry	1/4 recipe	278	4	37	4	2 1/2
Chicken Hungarian Goulash	1 1/2 cups	315	4	38	4	2 1/2
Roast Chicken and Vegetables	1/4 recipe	405	11	39	5	2 1/2
Chicken and Black Bean Burritos	1/6 recipe	255	3	40	3	2 1/2
SEAFOOD						
Seafood Dijon Fettuccini	1 1/3 cups	300	6	37	2	2 1/2
Seafood Pasta	1/6 recipe	301	5	38	2	2 1/2
BEEF AND PORK						
Swiss Steak with Rice	1 1/2 cups	316	6	36	4	2 1/2
Beef Hungarian Goulash (v)	1 1/2 cups	321	6	38	4	2 1/2
GROUND MEAT AND SAUSAGE						
Macaroni and Sausage Casserole	1/6 recipe	293	18	37	3	2 1/2
Chili Tamale Pie	1/6 recipe	254	4	39	5	2 1/2
Pasta Sea Shell Casserole	1 1/3 cups	270	5	39	3	2 1/2

*Carb Servings listed have been adjusted for fiber. In some recipes this resulted in no change. If the fiber is more than 5 grams, half of the grams of fiber are subtracted from the total grams of carbohydrate when figuring Exchanges and Carb Servings.

(v) = variation

One portion of the following recipes has 41–50 grams of carbohydrates and is counted as 3 Carb Servings.

	One Serving	Calories	Total Fat grams	Carbohydrate grams	Dietary Fiber grams	Carb Servings
MEATLESS ENTREES						
Eggplant Lasagna	1/10 recipe	270	5	41	3	3
Vegetable Lasagna	1/10 recipe	247	4	41	3	3
Macaroni and Cheese Casserole	1 1/2 cups	298	17	43	3	3
Pesto Linguini	1 cup	253	6	42	1	3
Harvest Primavera	1/5 recipe	241	2	47	4	3
Italian Curry Pasta	1 1/4 cups	260	3	49	5	3
POULTRY						
Patio Chicken and Rice	1/5 recipe	373	7	43	5	3
SEAFOOD						
Pasta with Clam Sauce	1/4 recipe	299	2	46	4	3

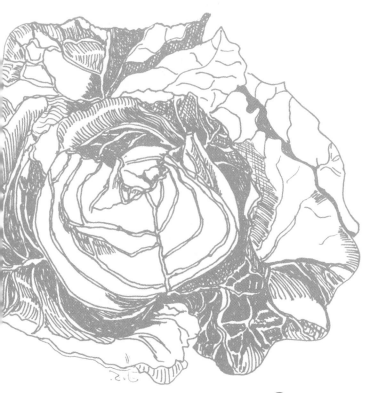

Measurements and Metric Conversions

Standard Measures

3 teaspoons	=	1 tablespoon
4 tablespoons	=	1/4 cup
8 tablespoons	=	1/2 cup
16 tablespoons	=	1 cup
1 cup	=	8 ounces, fluid
2 cups	=	1 pint
4 cups	=	1 quart
4 quarts	=	1 gallon
16 ounces	=	1 pound

Weights

U.S.		Metric
1 oz	=	28 g
2 oz	=	57 g
4 oz (1/4 lb)	=	114 g
6 oz	=	170 g
8 oz (1/2 lb)	=	227 g
12 oz (3/4 lb)	=	340 g
1 lb (16 oz)	=	454 g

Length

U.S.		Metric
1 inch	=	2.54 cm
8 inches	=	20 cm
9 inches	=	23 cm
13 inches	=	33 cm

Figures Based on

1 oz	=	28.35 g
1 lb	=	453.59 g
1 Tbsp	=	14.8 ml
1 cup	=	237 ml

Volume

U.S.		Metric
1/4 tsp	=	1 ml
1/2 tsp	=	2 ml
1 tsp	=	5 ml
2 tsp	=	10 ml
1 Tbsp	=	15 ml
1/4 cup (4 Tbsp)	=	60 ml
1/3 cup	=	80 ml
1/2 cup (8 Tbsp)	=	120 ml
2/3 cup	=	160 ml
3/4 cup	=	180 ml
1 cup (16 Tbsp)	=	240 ml
2 cups	=	480 ml
4 cups (1 quart)	=	950 ml

Temperatures

Fahrenheit		Celsius
325	=	165
350	=	175
375	=	190
400	=	205
425	=	220
450	=	230

Abbreviations

oz	=	ounce
lb	=	pound
tsp	=	teaspoon
Tbsp	=	tablespoon
qt	=	quart
g	=	grams
ml	=	milliliter
cm	=	centimeter
l	=	liter

Appetizers and Sauces

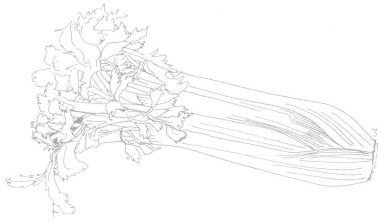

Small amounts of appetizers and sauces provide variety and fit well in a healthy diet. However, keep in mind that large amounts can contribute excessive calories. So, watch your portions!

Some of these recipes use the fat-free version of cream cheese, since the light version still has a fair amount of fat. Fat-free cream cheese is very acceptable in recipes when the predominant flavor is from other ingredients. The difference in saturated fat is: fat-free cream cheese has 0 grams saturated fat, while reduced-fat cream cheese has 3 grams of saturated fat for 2 tablespoons.

Cheese Sauce

A creamy sauce that's good on potatoes, broccoli, asparagus, or cauliflower.

Makes about 1 cup
8 servings

Each Serving
2 tablespoons

Carb Servings
0

Exchanges
1/2 fat-free milk

Nutrient Analysis
calories 40
total fat 1g
saturated fat 1g
cholesterol 6mg
sodium 72mg
total carbohydrate 3g
dietary fiber 0g
sugars 1g
protein 4g

1 cup fat-free milk, divided
2 tablespoons unbleached all-purpose flour
1/4 teaspoon salt (optional)
1/8 teaspoon ground black pepper
2 ounces reduced-fat sharp cheddar cheese,
    cut into small pieces

Combine 1/2 cup milk with flour in covered container and shake well to prevent lumps. Pour into a 4-cup glass measuring cup along with the rest of the milk and seasonings.

Cook in the microwave on high for 3–4 minutes, stirring with a wire whisk every 60 seconds or until bubbly and thickened. Add cheese and stir until melted.

VARIATION: *Dill Cheese Sauce*—Add 1 1/2 teaspoons of dried dill weed with seasonings.

Dijon Sauce

3 tablespoons light mayonnaise
2 tablespoons fat-free plain yogurt
2 teaspoons Dijon mustard
1 teaspoon honey or the equivalent in artificial sweetener

Combine all ingredients and mix well. Use as a dip or as a dressing.

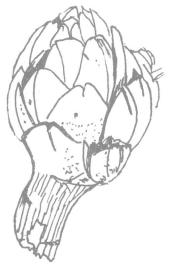

Try this sauce as a dip for raw cauliflower and zucchini slices or for cooked artichokes. This sauce is also good on sliced tomatoes or cucumbers.

Makes 6 tablespoons
6 servings

Each Serving
1 tablespoon

Carb Servings
0

Exchanges
1/2 fat

Nutrient Analysis
calories 26
total fat 2g
saturated fat 0g
cholesterol 0mg
sodium 110mg
total carbohydrate 2g
dietary fiber 0g
sugars 1g
protein 0g

Serve as a dip for raw vegetables such as jícama, celery, carrot sticks, and pepper slices.

Makes about 2 cups
16 servings

Each Serving
2 tablespoons

Carb Servings
0

Exchanges
1/2 starch

Nutrient Analysis
calories 32
total fat 1g
saturated fat 0g
cholesterol 2mg
sodium 89mg
total carbohydrate 5g
dietary fiber 1g
sugars 1g
protein 3g

Layered Black Bean Dip

1 can (15 ounces) black beans, drained and rinsed
1/4 teaspoon onion powder
1/4 teaspoon dried oregano
1/8 teaspoon garlic powder
1/8 teaspoon cayenne pepper
1/2 cup salsa, thick and chunky
1/2 cup fat-free sour cream
1/4 cup chopped green onions
2 ounces (1/2 cup) grated reduced-fat cheddar cheese

Mash beans, and mix with onion powder, dried oregano, garlic powder, and cayenne pepper. Spread on a serving dish.

Top with salsa, sour cream, green onions, and grated cheese.

Bean and Salsa Dip

1 can (16 ounces) fat-free refried beans
1/2 cup salsa, thick and chunky

Mix all ingredients in a microwave-safe bowl.

Cover, venting the lid, and cook on high until hot (about 1 minute), stirring a couple times during cooking.

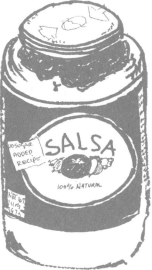

The salsa adds flavor to this dip. Serve with baked tortilla chips or raw veggies. Use a hot salsa if you choose.

Makes 2 cups
16 servings

Each Serving
2 tablespoons

Carb Servings
0

Exchanges
1 vegetable

Nutrient Analysis
calories 24
total fat 0g
saturated fat 0g
cholesterol 0mg
sodium 164mg
total carbohydrate 4g
dietary fiber 1g
sugars 0g
protein 1g

The cream cheese adds a little variety to this dip. Serve with celery sticks. For additional color, garnish with chopped green onion and chopped tomatoes.

Makes 2 cups
16 servings

Each Serving
2 tablespoons

Carb Servings
0

Exchanges
1 vegetable

Nutrient Analysis
calories 30
total fat 0g
saturated fat 0g
cholesterol 0mg
sodium 188mg
total carbohydrate 4g
dietary fiber 1g
sugars 1g
protein 2g

Bean and Cheese Dip

1 can (16 ounces) fat-free refried beans
1/2 cup (4 ounces) fat-free cream cheese
1/4 cup salsa, thick and chunky

Combine all ingredients in a microwave-safe bowl.

Cover, venting the lid, and cook on high until hot (about 1 minute), stirring a couple times during cooking.

Chili Cheese Dip

1 can (15 ounces) reduced-fat turkey chili with beans*
1/2 cup (4 ounces) fat-free cream cheese

Combine all ingredients in a microwave-safe bowl.

Cover, venting the lid, and cook on high until hot (about 1 minute), stirring a couple times during cooking.

Or choose a chili with no more than 8 grams of fat per 220 calories.

This dip is popular at parties. Watch your portion size, since the calories can easily add up.

Makes 2 cups
16 servings

Each Serving
2 tablespoons

Carb Servings
0

Exchanges
1/2 starch

Nutrient Analysis
calories 32
total fat 0g
saturated fat 0g
cholesterol 6mg
sodium 193mg
total carbohydrate 4g
dietary fiber 1g
sugars 1g
protein 3g

Use as a dip for vegetables or spread on cucumber or zucchini slices.

Makes 1 1/2 cups
12 servings

Each Serving
2 tablespoons

Carb Servings
0

Exchanges
1 lean meat

Nutrient Analysis
calories 26
total fat 0g
saturated fat 0g
cholesterol 0mg
sodium 130mg
total carbohydrate 2g
dietary fiber 0g
sugars 2g
protein 4g

Cream Cheese Spread

1 tub (8 ounces) fat-free cream cheese, at
   room temperature
1/2 cup fat-free sour cream
1 tablespoon dried onion
1 tablespoon dried parsley
1 teaspoon dried basil
1/4 teaspoon each: dried thyme and garlic powder
1/8 teaspoon ground black pepper

Combine all ingredients, and mix well.

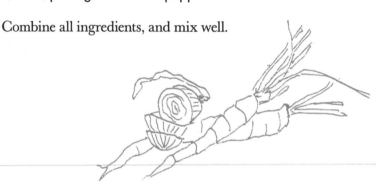

Cucumber Spread

1 tub (8 ounces) fat-free cream cheese, at
   room temperature
1 cup finely chopped cucumber, not peeled
6 green onions, minced
2 tablespoons fat-free sour cream
1/8 teaspoon ground black pepper

Combine all ingredients, and mix well.

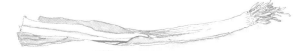

*Use as a spread on
cocktail bread, cucumber
slices, or celery sticks.*

Makes 2 cups
16 servings

Each Serving
2 tablespoons

Carb Servings
0

Exchanges
free

Nutrient Analysis
calories 18
total fat 0g
saturated fat 0g
cholesterol 0mg
sodium 90mg
total carbohydrate 2g
dietary fiber 0g
sugars 1g
protein 2g

This can be used as a party spread or at lunchtime on whole-grain bagels.

Makes 1 cup
8 servings

Each Serving
2 tablespoons

Carb Servings
0

Exchanges
1 lean meat

Nutrient Analysis
calories 40
total fat 1g
saturated fat 0g
cholesterol 1mg
sodium 202mg
total carbohydrate 1g
dietary fiber 0g
sugars 1g
protein 4g

Herbed Cream Cheese

1 tub (8 ounces) fat-free cream cheese, at
  room temperature
2 tablespoons light mayonnaise
1 teaspoon lemon juice
1 teaspoon chopped garlic
1/2 teaspoon onion powder
1/2 teaspoon Italian seasoning

Combine all ingredients, and mix well.

Serve spread on bagels, crackers, toast, cucumbers, zucchini, celery, and other crisp foods.

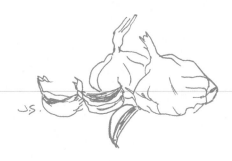

Pimento and Cheese Spread

1 jar (2 ounces) pimento, drained
4 ounces (1 cup) grated reduced-fat cheddar cheese
1/4 cup light mayonnaise
1/8 teaspoon garlic powder

Combine all ingredients and mix well.

For a hot appetizer, spread on French bread and broil until cheese is melted.

For a cold appetizer, arrange sliced vegetables and crackers on a platter around a bowl of the spread. Or make individual canapés by placing a small amount of the spread on vegetable slices such as zucchini and cucumber.

Simple and tasty, this spread can be used on vegetables, crackers, or bread.

Makes 1 cup
16 servings

Each Serving
1 tablespoon

Carb Servings
0

Exchanges
1/2 fat

Nutrient Analysis
calories 34
total fat 2g
saturated fat 1g
cholesterol 5mg
sodium 81mg
total carbohydrate 1g
dietary fiber 0g
sugars 0g
protein 2g

Makes 2 cups
16 servings

Each Serving
2 tablespoons

Carb Servings
0

Exchanges
1 lean meat

Nutrient Analysis
calories 34
total fat 0g
saturated fat 0g
cholesterol 8mg
sodium 176mg
total carbohydrate 1g
dietary fiber 0g
sugars 0g
protein 7g

Tuna Paté

1 tub (8 ounces) fat-free cream cheese, at room temperature
2 cans (6 ounces each) water-packed tuna, drained and flaked
2 tablespoons chili sauce
2 teaspoons dried parsley
1 teaspoon minced onion
4 drops Tabasco sauce

In a blender, combine all ingredients and blend until smooth.

Veggie Spread

1 tub (8 ounces) fat-free cream cheese, at
   room temperature
1/3 cup light mayonnaise
1 teaspoon dried dill weed
1 teaspoon dried parsley
1/2 teaspoon garlic powder
1/2 teaspoon dried basil
1 cup assorted finely chopped vegetables (such as bell
   peppers, carrots, celery, cauliflower, etc.)

Mix cream cheese, mayonnaise, dried dill weed, dried
parsley, garlic powder, and dried basil. Blend until
smooth.

Add chopped vegetables, reserving a few to sprinkle over
the top.

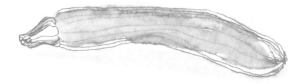

*This spread takes on the
flavor of the vegetables
that you add. Serve on
zucchini or cucumber slices
or use as a dip for carrots
and celery.*

Makes 2 cups
16 servings

Each Serving
2 tablespoons

Carb Servings
0

Exchanges
1 vegetable

Nutrient Analysis
calories 28
total fat 1g
saturated fat 0g
cholesterol 3mg
sodium 119mg
total carbohydrate 2g
dietary fiber 0g
sugars 0g
protein 2g

Breads

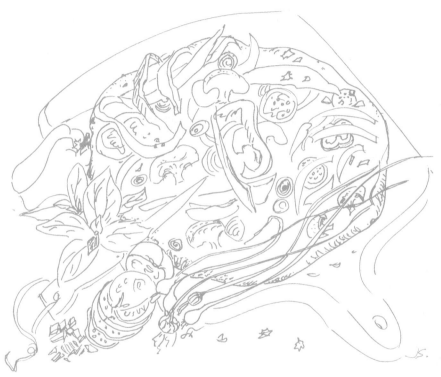

Breads and grains provide the foundation for a healthful diet. To save time when preparing some of the breads in this section, double the recipe and freeze half for later use. The sweeter breads have less sugar than most breakfast breads.

Makes 8 pancakes
4 servings

Each Serving
2 pancakes

Carb Servings
2

Exchanges
2 starch

Nutrient Analysis
calories 144
total fat 1g
saturated fat 0g
cholesterol 0mg
sodium 368mg
total carbohydrate 30g
dietary fiber 1g
sugars 9g
protein 4g

Apple Cider Pancakes

1/4 cup old-fashioned oats
1 cup pancake mix*
3/4 cup apple cider

Spray a griddle or skillet with nonstick cooking spray.

With a wire whisk, blend all ingredients until smooth.

Pour slightly less than 1/4 cup of batter per pancake on a hot griddle or skillet. Cook about 1 to 1 1/2 minutes on each side or until golden brown.

Look for no more than 3 grams of fat per 1/2 cup mix.

Banana Bread

1/2 cup granulated sugar
1/4 cup unsweetened applesauce
1/2 cup egg substitute (equal to 2 eggs)
1/4 cup fat-free milk
1 cup mashed banana
3/4 cup unbleached all-purpose flour
3/4 cup whole-wheat flour
1/2 cup oat bran
2 teaspoons baking powder
1/2 teaspoon ground cinnamon
1/4 teaspoon baking soda
1/4 teaspoon ground nutmeg
1/4 teaspoon salt (optional)

Preheat oven to 350 degrees. Spray an 8" × 8" pan with nonstick cooking spray.

In a large mixing bowl, combine sugar, applesauce, egg substitute, milk, and banana.

In a separate bowl, mix remaining ingredients. Add dry ingredients to the banana mixture. Stir just until flour is moistened. Pour into pan and bake for 50–55 minutes or until toothpick inserted in the center comes out clean.

NOTE: One serving is a good source of fiber.

Use ripe bananas in this fat-free bread. Serve as a breakfast bread or as a dessert with a dollop of fat-free whipped topping. Use an 8"× 8" pan instead of a loaf pan to cook more uniformly.

Makes 9 servings

Each Serving
1/9 recipe

Carb Servings
2

Exchanges
2 starch

Nutrient Analysis
calories 166
total fat 1g
saturated fat 0g
cholesterol 0mg
sodium 143mg
total carbohydrate 35g
dietary fiber 3g
sugars 15g
protein 5g

This is a variation of the popular buttermilk muffin recipe from my first book. It's very moist, high in fiber, and low in fat.

Makes 9 servings

Each Serving
1/9 recipe

Carb Servings
2

Exchanges
2 starch

Nutrient Analysis
calories 169
total fat 1g
saturated fat 0g
cholesterol 1mg
sodium 285mg
total carbohydrate 35g
dietary fiber 5g
sugars 15g
protein 5g

Buttermilk Bran Breakfast Squares

1/2 cup boiling water
1/2 cup All Bran cereal
1/4 cup egg substitute (equal to 1 egg)
1 cup low-fat buttermilk
1/2 cup granulated sugar
1/4 cup unsweetened applesauce
3/4 cup whole-wheat flour
1/2 cup unbleached all-purpose flour
1 teaspoon baking soda
1/2 teaspoon salt (optional)
1 cup Bran Buds or 100% Bran cereal

Preheat oven to 350 degrees. In a small bowl, pour boiling water over the All Bran cereal and let stand until softened.

In a large bowl, mix egg substitute, buttermilk, sugar, and applesauce. Add the All Bran/water mixture to the egg mixture. Stir in flours, baking soda, and salt (optional). Mix just until moistened. Stir in Bran Buds or 100% Bran cereal.

Pour into an 8" × 8" pan that has been sprayed with nonstick cooking spray. Bake for 55–60 minutes or until a toothpick inserted into the center comes out clean. Cut into 9 servings.

NOTE: One serving is an excellent source of fiber.

Carrot Muffins

1 3/4 cups unbleached all-purpose flour
3/4 cup granulated sugar
1/2 cup oat bran
1 teaspoon baking soda
1 teaspoon allspice
1/2 teaspoon salt (optional)
1/2 teaspoon baking powder
2 jars (6 ounces each) pureed carrots (baby food type)
1/2 cup egg substitute (equal to 2 eggs)
1/2 cup unsweetened applesauce
1/2 cup seedless raisins
1 teaspoon vanilla extract

Preheat oven to 350 degrees. Spray muffin tins with nonstick cooking spray.

In a medium bowl, combine flour, sugar, oat bran, baking soda, allspice, salt (optional), and baking powder.

In a larger bowl, mix carrots with remaining ingredients until well blended. Stir flour mixture into carrot mixture just until flour is moistened. Spoon batter into muffin tins. Bake for 30 minutes or until toothpick inserted in the center comes out clean.

These muffins have no added fat and taste great. Serve for breakfast or as a snack.

Makes 12 servings

Each Serving
1 muffin

Carb Servings
2 1/2

Exchanges
2 1/2 starch

Nutrient Analysis
calories 163
total fat 1g
saturated fat 0g
cholesterol 0mg
sodium 138mg
total carbohydrate 36g
dietary fiber 1g
sugars 16g
protein 4g

Makes 16 slices

Each Serving
1 slice

Carb Servings
2

Exchanges
2 starch

Nutrient Analysis
calories 156
total fat 2g
saturated fat 0g
cholesterol 0mg
sodium 86mg
total carbohydrate 32g
dietary fiber 1g
sugars 18g
protein 3g

Date Nut Bread

5 ounces dates, chopped (about 1 cup)
1 teaspoon baking soda
1 cup hot coffee
1 cup granulated sugar
1/4 cup egg substitute (equal to 1 egg)
1 tablespoon canola oil
1 teaspoon vanilla
1/8 teaspoon salt (optional)
2 cups unbleached all-purpose flour
1/2 cup chopped walnuts

Preheat oven to 350 degrees. Mix dates with baking soda and coffee. Set aside to cool.

Mix in sugar, egg substitute, canola oil, vanilla, and salt (optional). Add flour and stir just until flour is moistened. Fold in nuts.

Pour into a 9" × 5" × 3" loaf pan that has been sprayed with nonstick cooking spray. Bake for 55–60 minutes or until a toothpick inserted in the center comes out clean.

Pineapple Bread

3/4 cup unbleached all-purpose flour
3/4 cup whole-wheat flour
1/2 cup oat bran
1/2 cup brown sugar
2 teaspoons baking powder
1/2 teaspoon cinnamon
1/2 teaspoon salt (optional)
1/2 teaspoon baking soda
1 can (8 ounces) crushed pineapple (in juice), not drained
1/2 cup egg substitute (equal to 2 eggs)
1/4 cup unsweetened applesauce

Preheat oven to 350 degrees. Spray an 8" × 8" pan with nonstick cooking spray.

Blend dry ingredients. Mix remaining ingredients in a separate bowl. Stir into flour mixture just until flour is moistened. Pour into pan.

Bake 40–45 minutes, or until a toothpick inserted in the center comes out clean.

This pineapple bread has no added fat and is a good choice for breakfast or dessert. Use an 8" × 8" pan instead of a loaf pan to cook more uniformly. This is a heavy-textured bread compared to most quick breads.

Makes 9 servings

Each Serving
1/9 recipe

Carb Servings
2

Exchanges
2 starch

Nutrient Analysis
calories 158
total fat 1g
saturated fat 0g
cholesterol 0mg
sodium 179mg
total carbohydrate 33g
dietary fiber 2g
sugars 15g
protein 5g

Makes 9 servings

Each Serving
1/9 recipe

Carb Servings
2 1/2

Exchanges
2 1/2 starch

Nutrient Analysis
calories 187
total fat 1g
saturated fat 0g
cholesterol 0mg
sodium 186mg
total carbohydrate 40g
dietary fiber 3g
sugars 17g
protein 5g

Pumpkin Bread

1 cup unbleached all-purpose flour
3/4 cup whole-wheat flour
3/4 cup granulated sugar
1/2 cup oat bran
1 teaspoon baking soda
1/2 teaspoon salt (optional)
1/2 teaspoon baking powder
1/2 teaspoon allspice
1/2 teaspoon cinnamon
1/2 teaspoon ground cloves
1 cup canned pumpkin
1/2 cup egg substitute (equal to 2 eggs)
1/2 cup unsweetened applesauce
1 teaspoon vanilla extract

Preheat oven to 350 degrees. Spray an 8" × 8" pan with nonstick cooking spray.

In a medium bowl, combine dry ingredients. In a larger bowl, mix pumpkin with remaining ingredients until well blended. Stir flour mixture into pumpkin mixture just until flour is moistened. Pour into pan.

Bake for 55–60 minutes or until toothpick inserted in the center comes out clean.

NOTE: One serving is a good source of fiber.

Bread Sticks

1 loaf (1 pound) frozen whole-wheat bread dough,
  thawed according to package directions
1/4 cup egg substitute (equal to 1 egg)

OPTIONAL INGREDIENTS:
Before baking, sprinkle with 1 tsp of one of the following:
  caraway seeds
  poppy seeds
  sesame seeds
  grated Parmesan cheese
  Italian seasoning

Preheat oven to 375 degrees. Lightly coat a baking sheet
with nonstick cooking spray.

Cut bread dough into 12 equal pieces. Stretch and shape
each piece into a 7" rope. Place on baking sheet. Brush
with egg.

Sprinkle with optional ingredients if desired. Set aside to
rise in a warm, draft-free location until doubled in size,
about 1 hour.

Bake 10 minutes, until golden brown. Immediately
remove bread sticks from baking sheet.

*If you like bread sticks
but don't want to take the
time to make them from
scratch, try this simple
recipe that uses frozen
bread dough. To save
time, thaw a loaf in the
refrigerator overnight.*

**Makes 12 bread
sticks**

Each Serving
1 bread stick

Carb Servings
1

Exchanges
1 starch
1/2 fat

Nutrient Analysis
calories 106
total fat 3g
saturated fat 0g
cholesterol 0mg
sodium 220mg
total carbohydrate 18g
dietary fiber 2g
sugars 2g
protein 5g

These are quick to prepare and taste so good. It's hard to believe they are low in fat. Also, you can serve these as a dessert shortcake with sliced fruit and light whipped topping.

Makes 8 biscuits

Each Serving
1 biscuit

Carb Servings
2

Exchanges
2 starch

Nutrient Analysis
calories 165
total fat 4g
saturated fat 0g
cholesterol 1mg
sodium 152mg
total carbohydrate 28g
dietary fiber 1g
sugars 3g
protein 5g

Drop Biscuits

1 1/2 cups unbleached all-purpose flour
1/2 cup whole-wheat flour
1 tablespoon granulated sugar
1 tablespoon baking powder
1/4 teaspoon salt (optional)
1 cup fat-free milk
2 tablespoons canola oil

Preheat oven to 400 degrees. Spray a baking sheet with nonstick cooking spray.

Mix dry ingredients. Gradually stir in milk and oil, mixing with a fork until the mixture leaves the sides of the bowl.

Drop by spoonfuls onto the baking sheet, making 8 biscuits. Bake for 15 minutes or until golden brown.

OPTIONAL TOPPINGS: Sprinkle with grated Parmesan cheese and/or Italian seasoning before baking.

VARIATION A: *Traditional Biscuits*–Add an additional 1–2 tablespoons of flour so that the dough is firm enough to handle. Divide dough into 8 pieces and shape into 8 biscuits. Bake as for drop biscuits.

VARIATION B: *Biscuit Wedges*–Add an additional 1–2 tablespoons of flour so that the dough is firm enough to handle. Divide dough into 2 pieces and pat out to form two flat circles, about 6" in diameter, on the baking sheet. Score with a knife to form 8 wedges each. Bake for 15–20 minutes. Top each wedge with 1 teaspoon sugar-free jam or jelly (spreadable fruit) before serving.

Variations A & B

Makes 8 biscuits

Each Serving
1 biscuit

Carb Servings
2

Exchanges
2 starch

**Variation A
Nutrient Analysis**
calories 169
total fat 4g
saturated fat 0g
cholesterol 1mg
sodium 152mg
total carbohydrate 28g
dietary fiber 1g
sugars 3g
protein 5g

**Variation B
Nutrient Analysis**
calories 185
total fat 4g
saturated fat 0g
cholesterol 1mg
sodium 152mg
total carbohydrate 32g
dietary fiber 1g
sugars 7g
protein 5g

Focaccia Cheese Bread

1 pound loaf whole-wheat Focaccia bread
2 ounces reduced-fat sharp cheddar cheese, cut into
   small cubes
1/2 tablespoon pesto sauce or 1 teaspoon olive oil and
   1 teaspoon dried basil

Makes 16 servings

Preheat oven to 350 degrees.

Each Serving
1/16 loaf

Place bread on a baking sheet that has been sprayed with nonstick cooking spray. Poke cheese into the top of the bread. Brush with pesto sauce or olive oil and basil.

Carb Servings
1

Bake for 15–20 minutes or until golden brown.

Exchanges
1 starch

NOTE: One serving is a good source of fiber.

Nutrient Analysis
calories 87
total fat 2g
saturated fat 1g
cholesterol 3mg
sodium 212mg
total carbohydrate 13g
dietary fiber 3g
sugars 1g
protein 4g

Focaccia Veggie Bread

1 pound loaf whole-wheat Focaccia bread
1 teaspoon olive oil
1 teaspoon Italian seasoning
1 green onion, chopped
1/4 cup diced green bell pepper
1/2 tablespoon grated Parmesan cheese

Preheat oven to 350 degrees.

Place bread on a baking sheet that has been sprayed with nonstick cooking spray.

Brush bread top with olive oil and sprinkle with Italian seasoning. Press onion and pepper into the top of the bread. Sprinkle with cheese.

Bake for 15–20 minutes or until golden brown.

NOTE: One serving is a good source of fiber.

This store-bought Focaccia bread takes on a delicious flavor with the addition of chopped fresh vegetables.

Makes 16 servings

Each Serving
1/16 loaf

Carb Servings
1

Exchanges
1 starch

Nutrient Analysis
calories 77
total fat 2g
saturated fat 0g
cholesterol 0mg
sodium 183mg
total carbohydrate 13g
dietary fiber 3g
sugars 1g
protein 3g

Makes 9 servings

Each Serving
1/9 recipe

Carb Servings
1 1/2

Exchanges
1 1/2 starch
1 fat

Nutrient Analysis
calories 169
total fat 6g
saturated fat 1g
cholesterol 5mg
sodium 160mg
total carbohydrate 22g
dietary fiber 2g
sugars 3g
protein 6g

Mexican Cornbread

1 can (15 ounces) cream style corn*
1/2 cup egg substitute (equal to 2 eggs)
1 cup yellow cornmeal
3/4 cup fat-free milk
3 tablespoons canola oil
1/2 teaspoon baking soda
1/2 teaspoon salt (optional)
1 can (4 ounces) diced green chiles
2 ounces (1/2 cup) grated reduced-fat cheddar cheese

Preheat oven to 400 degrees.

Mix all ingredients in a medium bowl. Pour into an 8" × 8" pan that has been sprayed with nonstick cooking spray.

Bake for 35–40 minutes or until a toothpick inserted in the center comes out clean.

Sodium is figured for no added salt.

Soups and Stews

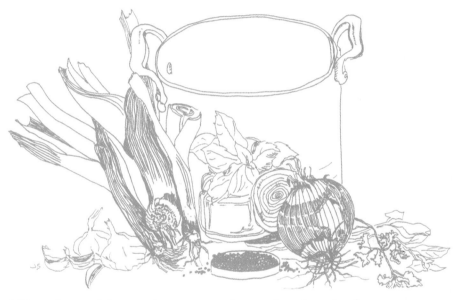

There's nothing quite as good as a hot bowl of soup on a cold winter day. Soups are good low-fat choices, especially if you use fat-free broth. Skim the fat from both, whether homemade or canned, to make it fat free. Refrigerate soups for several hours, and the fat will harden and can be easily removed. Some of the recipes in this section are a complete meal or can become a complete meal by the addition of a bread or a salad. Plan on having the leftovers for lunch.

Try this served in a mug as an accompaniment to a sandwich on a cold winter day or as a hot drink in the evening. Chicken or vegetable broth can be substituted for beef.

Makes 1 serving

Each Serving
1 cup

Carb Servings
0

Exchanges
free

Nutrient Analysis
calories 19
total fat 0g
saturated fat 0g
cholesterol 0mg
sodium 379mg
total carbohydrate 3g
dietary fiber 0g
sugars 3g
protein 2g

Sherried Broth

1 cup fat-free beef broth*
2 tablespoons dry sherry

Mix ingredients in a microwave-safe mug. Heat on high in microwave for 2–3 minutes or until hot.

Sodium is figured for reduced sodium.

Tortilla Soup

4 cups fat-free chicken broth*
1 medium tomato, chopped
4 green onions, chopped
3 corn tortillas, cut into eighths

In a medium saucepan, mix broth, tomato, and onion.
Cover and bring to a boil. Reduce heat to low.

Add tortillas and simmer, covered, for 15 minutes.

Sodium is figured for reduced sodium.

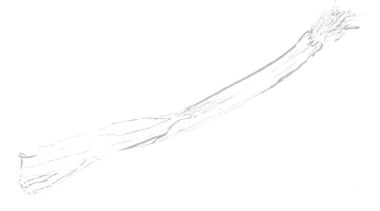

*This is a great first course
to a Mexican meal.
It is also a good choice
for lunch.*

Makes 5 cups
4 servings

Each Serving
1 1/4 cups

Carb Servings
1

Exchanges
1/2 starch
1 vegetable

Nutrient Analysis
calories 79
total fat 1g
saturated fat 0g
cholesterol 0mg
sodium 413mg
total carbohydrate 14g
dietary fiber 1g
sugars 3g
protein 4g

Serve this hot soup in a mug. It is good served with a sandwich or as a hot drink on a cold winter day.

Makes 2 cups
2 servings

Each Serving
1 cup

Carb Servings
1/2

Exchanges
1 vegetable

Nutrient Analysis
calories 41
total fat 0g
saturated fat 0g
cholesterol 0mg
sodium 200mg
total carbohydrate 7g
dietary fiber 2g
sugars 4g
protein 2g

Spiced Tomato Broth

1 cup tomato juice*
1 cup fat-free beef broth*
3 black peppercorns
2 whole cloves
1/2 bay leaf
1 tablespoon lemon juice

Mix all ingredients in a saucepan. Cover and heat to boiling.

Reduce heat to low and simmer for 10 minutes. Discard peppercorns, cloves, and bay leaf before serving.

Sodium is figured for no added salt/reduced sodium.

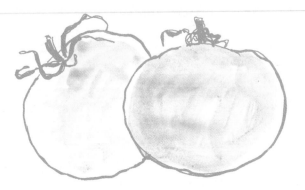

Black Bean Soup

1 cup chopped onion
3/4 cup chopped celery
2 teaspoons chopped garlic
1 1/2 cups fat-free beef broth*
2 cans (15 ounces each) black beans, drained and rinsed
1/2 cup salsa, thick and chunky
1 1/2 teaspoons ground cumin
1/2 teaspoon onion powder
1/4 teaspoon dried oregano

Combine all ingredients in a saucepan.

Cover and simmer for 20–25 minutes or until vegetables are tender.

NOTE: One serving is an excellent source of fiber.

Sodium is figured for reduced sodium.

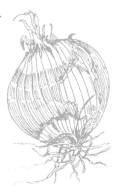

Serve this thick soup for a quick lunch.

Makes 5 cups
4 servings

Each Serving
1 1/4 cups

Carb Servings**
2

Exchanges**
1 1/2 starch
1 vegetable
1 lean meat

Nutrient Analysis
calories 171
total fat 1g
saturated fat 0g
cholesterol 0mg
sodium 391mg
total carbohydrate 30g
dietary fiber 6g
sugars 1g
protein 11g

**Half of the grams of fiber have been subtracted from the grams of total carbohydrate when figuring Carb Servings and Exchanges.*

This is an excellent recipe for cabbage. It has a wonderful flavor and a creamy texture.

Makes 8 cups
5 servings

Each Serving
1 1/2 cups

Carb Servings
1

Exchanges
1/2 starch
1 vegetable
2 lean meat

Nutrient Analysis
calories 155
total fat 4g
saturated fat 1g
cholesterol 29mg
sodium 640mg
total carbohydrate 15g
dietary fiber 2g
sugars 3g
protein 14g

Creamy Cabbage Soup

1 small head of cabbage (about 1 pound)
3/4 cup chopped onion
8 ounces reduced-fat turkey smoked sausage (Polish kielbasa type), sliced
4 cups fat-free chicken broth*
3/4 cup fat-free milk
1/4 cup unbleached all-purpose flour
1/8 teaspoon ground black pepper

Chop cabbage. Combine cabbage, onion, sausage, and chicken broth in a large saucepan. Simmer until vegetables are tender.

Combine milk with flour in covered container and shake well to prevent lumps. Stir into soup along with pepper. Heat until bubbly.

Sodium is figured for reduced sodium.

Garden Minestrone

1 pound extra-lean ground beef or ground turkey (7% fat)
6 cups fat-free beef broth*
2 cups chopped cabbage
1 can (14.5 ounces) diced tomatoes, not drained*
1 can (14.5 ounces) green beans, not drained*
1 cup sliced carrots
1 cup sliced zucchini
1 cup uncooked elbow macaroni
2 tablespoons dried chopped onion
2 tablespoons dried parsley
1 tablespoon chopped garlic
1 teaspoon dried basil
1/2 teaspoon dried oregano
1/4 teaspoon ground black pepper

Brown meat in a 4-quart kettle that has been sprayed with nonstick cooking spray.

Add remaining ingredients and simmer until vegetables are tender, about 20 minutes.

NOTE: One serving is an excellent source of fiber.

Sodium is figured for no-added salt/reduced sodium.

This is a colorful, hearty soup that can be enjoyed year-round. Take advantage of summer vegetables and serve this for a quick supper. You can also make this soup without the ground meat. Plan on freezing leftovers for another meal.

Makes 9 cups
6 servings

Each Serving
1 1/2 cups

Carb Servings
1 1/2

Exchanges
1 starch
2 vegetable
3 lean meat

Nutrient Analysis
calories 245
total fat 6g
saturated fat 2g
cholesterol 46mg
sodium 465mg
total carbohydrate 25g
dietary fiber 5g
sugars 8g
protein 21g

This is a hearty soup is a complete meal. You can substitute quick-cooking barley, rice, or noodles for the orzo. Orzo is pasta that looks like rice. This recipe makes a large amount, so you can have leftovers for lunch or freeze for another meal.

Makes 11 cups
7 servings

Each Serving
about 1 1/2 cups

Carb Servings
2

Exchanges
1 starch
3 vegetable
2 lean meat

Nutrient Analysis
calories 262
total fat 5g
saturated fat 2g
cholesterol 40mg
sodium 387mg
total carbohydrate 33g
dietary fiber 5g
sugars 7g
protein 20g

Venus de Milo Soup

1 pound extra-lean ground beef or ground turkey (7% fat)
3 cups water
5 cups fat-free beef broth*
1 large onion, chopped
1 package (16 ounces) frozen mixed vegetables
1 can (14.5 ounces) stewed tomatoes, not drained*
1 can (8 ounces) tomato sauce*
1/4 teaspoon salt (optional)
1/8 teaspoon ground black pepper
3/4 cup uncooked orzo or quick-cooking barley
1 tablespoon grated Parmesan cheese

In a large pot that has been sprayed with nonstick cooking spray, brown meat. Add all but the orzo and Parmesan cheese.

Bring to a boil. Reduce heat to low, cover, and simmer for 20–25 minutes. Add orzo and cook for 15 minutes.

Serve with a sprinkling of Parmesan cheese.

NOTE: One serving is an excellent source of fiber.

Sodium is figured for no-added salt/reduced sodium.

Oven Beef Stew

2 pounds round steak, cut into cubes
3/4 cup chopped onion
1 stalk celery, sliced
2 medium potatoes, not peeled, cubed (14 ounces)
2 carrots, sliced
2 tablespoons tapioca
2 tablespoons dried parsley
1/2 teaspoon dried oregano
1/2 teaspoon salt (optional)
1/4 teaspoon garlic powder
1/8 teaspoon ground black pepper
1 bay leaf
1 1/2 cups tomato juice*
1 cup water

Preheat oven to 325 degrees. Mix all ingredients in a 4-quart Dutch oven.

Cover and bake for 2 1/2 hours.

NOTE: One serving is a good source of fiber.

Sodium is figured for no added salt.

This recipe may take a while to cook, but it doesn't require any attention once it's in the oven. This is a good dish to make on a Saturday afternoon and then have the leftovers during the week.

Makes 8 cups
8 servings

Each Serving
1 cup

Carb Servings
1 1/2

Exchanges
1 starch
1 vegetable
3 lean meat

Nutrient Analysis
calories 220
total fat 4g
saturated fat 1g
cholesterol 55mg
sodium 87mg
total carbohydrate 23g
dietary fiber 3g
sugars 5g
protein 23g

This hearty stew takes just minutes to put together and is a good choice for a quick supper.

Makes 11 cups
11 servings

Each Serving
1 cup

Carb Servings
2 1/2

Exchanges
2 starch
1 vegetable
1 lean meat

Nutrient Analysis
calories 228
total fat 2g
saturated fat 1g
cholesterol 13mg
sodium 195mg
total carbohydrate 40g
dietary fiber 5g
sugars 3g
protein 13g

Sausage and Lentil Stew

2 cups lentils
5 1/2 cups water
1 1/2 cups chopped onion
4 medium potatoes, not peeled, cubed (20 ounces)
1 1/2 cups sliced carrots
4 teaspoons chopped garlic
8 ounces reduced-fat turkey smoked sausage (Polish kielbasa type), sliced

Rinse lentils. In a 4-quart saucepan, mix all ingredients.

Bring to a boil, then reduce heat and simmer for 30 minutes or until lentils are tender.

NOTE: One serving is an excellent source of fiber.

Green Chile Pork Stew

1 pound boneless pork tenderloin
3/4 cup chopped onion
3/4 cup sliced celery
2 carrots, sliced
2 medium potatoes, not peeled, cubed (14 ounces)
1 can (7 ounces) diced green chiles
2 teaspoons chopped garlic
1 cup fat-free chicken broth*
1 cup water (or enough to cover)
2 tablespoons cornstarch
1/4 cup water
salsa, thick and chunky (optional)

Cut pork into 1 1/2 inch cubes. In a 3-quart saucepan, mix pork with the vegetables and chicken broth. Add water to cover. Cover and simmer about 45 minutes.

Mix cornstarch with remaining water. Add to stew and cook until bubbly. Serve as is or topped with a spoonful of salsa.

NOTE: One serving is a good source of fiber.

Sodium is figured for reduced sodium.

A great dish for a cold winter day.

Makes 7 1/2 cups
5 servings

Each Serving
1 1/2 cups

Carb Servings
2 1/2

Exchanges
1 1/2 starch
2 vegetable
2 lean meat

Nutrient Analysis
calories 269
total fat 4g
saturated fat 1g
cholesterol 52mg
sodium 187mg
total carbohydrate 37g
dietary fiber 4g
sugars 6g
protein 23g

If you like seafood and tomatoes, you'll like this Southern stew. Serve with a whole-grain bread to complete the meal.

Makes 8 cups
5 servings

Each Serving
about 1 1/2 cups

Carb Servings
1

Exchanges
2 vegetable
3 lean meat

Nutrient Analysis
calories 163
total fat 2g
saturated fat 0g
cholesterol 33mg
sodium 237mg
total carbohydrate 14g
dietary fiber 2g
sugars 5g
protein 23g

Seafood Gumbo

1 can (28 ounces) diced tomatoes, not drained*
1/2 cup chopped onion
1 package (8 ounces) frozen okra or 1 1/2 cups sliced celery
2 cups fat-free chicken or beef broth*
1 teaspoon chopped garlic
1 teaspoon paprika
1/8 teaspoon cayenne pepper
1 drop Tabasco sauce
3 tablespoons unbleached all-purpose flour
1/2 cup water
1 pound seafood such as firm fish fillets, scallops, and/or shelled and deveined shrimp

In a medium saucepan, mix vegetables, broth, and seasonings. Simmer, covered, until vegetables are tender.

Combine flour and water in a covered container and shake well to prevent lumps. Add to simmering vegetables and cook until bubbly. Add seafood and continue to cook until seafood is done.

Sodium is figured for no added salt/reduced sodium.

Chicken Chili

1/2 pound skinless, boneless chicken breasts
3/4 cup chopped onion
2 teaspoons chopped garlic
2 cans (15 ounces each) kidney beans, drained and rinsed
1 can (14.5 ounces) diced tomatoes, not drained*
1 can (4 ounces) diced green chiles
1 cup water
1 tablespoon dried cilantro
2 teaspoons chili powder
1/2 teaspoon ground cumin

Cut chicken into bite-size pieces.

Brown chicken in a saucepan that has been sprayed with nonstick cooking spray. Add remaining ingredients.

Cover and simmer for 30 minutes or until chicken is tender.

NOTE: One serving is an excellent source of fiber.

Sodium is figured for no added salt.

Chili lovers will enjoy this thick chili. It is so simple and tasty.

Makes 6 cups
5 servings

Each Serving
1 1/4 cups

Carb Servings**
2

Exchanges**
1 1/2 starch
1 vegetable
2 lean meat

Nutrient Analysis
calories 236
total fat 2g
saturated fat 0g
cholesterol 28mg
sodium 64mg
total carbohydrate 33g
dietary fiber 10g
sugars 3g
protein 21g

**Half of the grams of fiber have been subtracted from the grams of total carbohydrate when figuring Carb Servings and Exchanges.

Makes 8 cups
5 servings

Each Serving
about 1 1/2 cups

Carb Servings
1 1/2

Exchanges
1 starch
1 vegetable
3 lean meat

Nutrient Analysis
calories 223
total fat 3g
saturated fat 1g
cholesterol 49mg
sodium 249mg
total carbohydrate 25g
dietary fiber 2g
sugars 2g
protein 25g

Chicken Pasta Stew

1 pound skinless, boneless chicken breasts,
   cut into 1-inch pieces
3/4 cup chopped onion
3/4 cup sliced celery
1 can (7 ounces) diced green chiles
2 teaspoons chopped garlic
2 cups fat-free chicken broth*
1 cup water
4 ounces egg noodles, "no yolk" type (2 cups uncooked)
1 1/2 cups frozen mixed peas and carrots

In a 3-quart saucepan, mix chicken with all but the noodles and mixed vegetables. Simmer, covered, for 15 minutes.

Add remaining ingredients. Simmer, uncovered, 15 minutes or until noodles are tender.

Sodium is figured for reduced sodium.

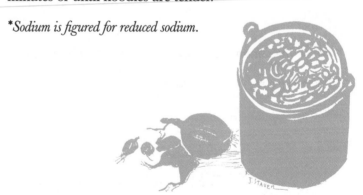

Chicken Soup

4 ounces skinless, boneless chicken breasts,
  cut into bite-size pieces
3 cups fat-free chicken broth*
2 cups water
2/3 cup sliced celery
1/2 cup sliced carrot
1/4 cup chopped onion
1 tablespoon dried parsley
1/2 cup frozen peas
2 ounces medium-size seashell pasta (1 cup uncooked)

In a medium saucepan, combine chicken with broth, water, celery, carrots, onion, and parsley.

Simmer, covered, until vegetables are soft. Add peas and pasta. Cook about 15 minutes or until pasta is tender.

Sodium is figured for reduced sodium.

This will remind you of real homemade chicken soup but without all the work. It's great on a cold winter day with a hot roll.

Makes 6 cups
4 servings

Each Serving
1 1/2 cups

Carb Servings
1

Exchanges
1 starch
1 vegetable
1 lean meat

Nutrient Analysis
calories 142
total fat 1g
saturated fat 0g
cholesterol 17mg
sodium 377mg
total carbohydrate 18g
dietary fiber 2g
sugars 5g
protein 14g

Vegetables

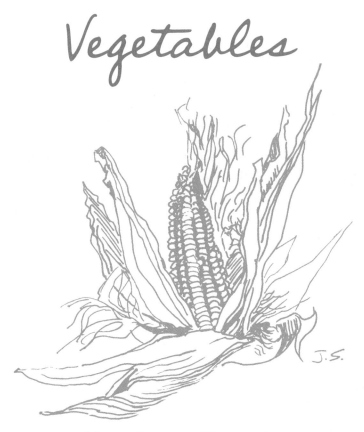

J.S.

The recipes in this section provide creative ways to prepare vegetables for the whole family to enjoy. Some are prepared in the microwave, some are barbecued, and some are cooked on the stove. All are quick to prepare.

Using the microwave to cook fresh vegetables is simple and brings out their good flavor. It is my favorite method for cooking vegetables. Consult a microwave cookbook for a table of basic cooking times.

Makes 2 cups
4 servings

Each Serving
1/2 cup

Carb Servings
0

Exchanges
1 vegetable

Nutrient Analysis
calories 35
total fat 2g
saturated fat 0mg
total cholesterol 0mg
sodium 56mg
total carbohydrate 3g
dietary fiber 1g
sugars 1g
protein 1g

Cucumbers with Dill Yogurt

2 tablespoons fat-free plain yogurt
2 tablespoons light mayonnaise
1/2 teaspoon dried dill weed
1/8 teaspoon salt (optional)
2 cups sliced cucumber, not peeled

Mix yogurt, mayonnaise, and seasonings. Gently toss with cucumbers.

Refrigerate to chill thoroughly.

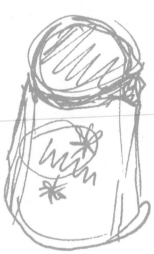

Cucumbers with Onions and Sour Cream

2 tablespoons fat-free sour cream
1 1/2 cups sliced cucumber, not peeled
1/2 red onion, sliced very thin and cut into quarters
  (1/2 cup)
1/8 teaspoon ground black pepper
1/8 teaspoon salt (optional)

Mix sour cream, cucumber, and onion. Add seasonings.

Refrigerate to chill thoroughly.

The combination of onions with cucumbers seems to be a favorite for many. The red onions add to the flavor as well as to the eye appeal of this dish. Sweet onions can be substituted for red onions.

Makes 2 cups
4 servings

Each Serving
1/2 cup

Carb Servings
0

Exchanges
free

Nutrient Analysis
calories 18
total fat 0g
saturated fat 0mg
cholesterol 0mg
sodium 1mg
total carbohydrate 4g
dietary fiber 1g
sugars 1g
protein 1g

Makes 2 cups
4 servings

Each Serving
1/2 cup

Carb Servings
1/2

Exchanges
1 vegetable

Nutrient Analysis
calories 35
total fat 1g
saturated fat 0mg
cholesterol 1mg
sodium 23mg
total carbohydrate 6g
dietary fiber 1g
sugars 2g
protein 1g

Tomatoes with Yogurt Dressing

1 tablespoon fat-free plain yogurt
1 tablespoon light mayonnaise
1/8 teaspoon garlic powder
1/8 teaspoon dried basil
1/8 teaspoon salt (optional)
2 cups chopped tomato

Mix yogurt, mayonnaise, and seasonings. Gently toss with tomatoes.

Refrigerate to thoroughly chill.

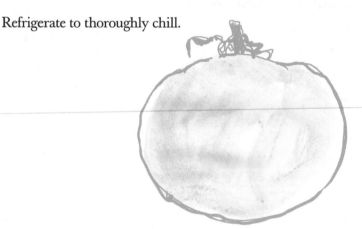

Barbecued Corn on the Cob

4 ears of corn

Start the barbecue. When hot, place unshucked corn directly on grill over high heat. Close hood and cook for 15 minutes, turning corn several times while cooking.

Remove corn and let sit until cool enough to handle. Pull down husks, and use as a handle.

NOTE: One serving is a good source of fiber.

This is an excellent way to prepare fresh corn on the barbecue, and it is so easy. The outside of the husks will blacken slightly, but the corn will be excellent. Serve this with any barbecued meat.

Makes 4 servings

Each Serving
1 ear of corn

Carb Servings
2

Exchanges
2 starch

Nutrient Analysis
calories 136
total fat 1g
saturated fat 0mg
cholesterol 0mg
sodium 5mg
total carbohydrate 28g
dietary fiber 3g
sugars 6g
protein 4g

Try these vegetables threaded on a skewer and barbecued. They are a great accompaniment to any barbecued meat. To prevent wooden skewers from burning, soak them in water for 10 minutes before using. This also works well with the addition of pineapple chunks.

Makes 4 servings

Each Serving
1/4 recipe

Carb Servings
0

Exchanges
1 vegetable

Nutrient Analysis
calories 23
total fat 0g
saturated fat 0mg
cholesterol 0mg
sodium 2mg
total carbohydrate 5g
dietary fiber 1g
sugars 2g
protein 1g

Barbecued Vegetable Kabobs

2 cups fresh vegetables, cut into bite-size pieces, such as bell peppers (red, yellow, green), whole mushroom caps, zucchini, and summer squash

Start the barbecue. Thread vegetables on skewers.

When the grill is hot, place skewers on the grill. Cover and cook for 10 minutes, turning halfway through cooking time.

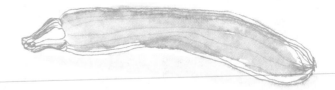

Barbecued Zucchini

2 small zucchini (about 5" long)
1/4 teaspoon Italian seasoning

Start the barbecue grill. Slice the zucchini in half, lengthwise.

When the barbecue is hot, place zucchini on the grill. Sprinkle with Italian seasoning. Close the hood and cook the zucchini 15–20 minutes, turning over halfway through cooking.

The flavor of this barbecued zucchini is so good, even people who don't like zucchini will like this recipe.

Makes 4 servings

_____

Each Serving
1/2 zucchini

Carb Servings
0

Exchanges
free

Nutrient Analysis
calories 12
total fat 0g
saturated fat 0mg
cholesterol 0mg
sodium 2mg
total carbohydrate 2g
dietary fiber 1g
sugars 1g
protein 1g

This is a simple and delicious way to prepare eggplant.

Makes 4 servings

Each Serving
1/4 recipe

Carb Servings
1/2

Exchanges
1 vegetable
1 fat

Nutrient Analysis
calories 62
total fat 3g
saturated fat 1mg
cholesterol 1mg
sodium 32mg
total carbohydrate 7g
dietary fiber 0g
sugars 1g
protein 2g

Grilled Eggplant

1 small eggplant (about 1 pound), not peeled
2 teaspoons olive oil
1/4 teaspoon garlic powder
1/8 teaspoon salt (optional)
1 tablespoon grated Parmesan cheese

Cut eggplant into slices 3/4 inch thick. Brush both sides with olive oil. Proceed with either method listed below.

STOVE TOP: Spray a large skillet or griddle with nonstick cooking spray. Place eggplant on the hot griddle and sprinkle with garlic powder and salt (optional). Cook about 4 minutes on each side or until tender. Remove from griddle and sprinkle with Parmesan cheese before serving.

BARBECUE: *Spray a piece of aluminum foil, large enough to hold the slices, with nonstick cooking spray and place on the barbecue grill. Start the barbecue. When hot, place eggplant slices on aluminum foil. Sprinkle with garlic powder and salt (optional). Close the hood and cook the eggplant 8 minutes, turning slices over halfway through cooking time. Remove from barbecue and sprinkle with Parmesan cheese before serving.

Nonstick cooking spray is flammable. Do not spray near open flame or heated surfaces.

Grilled Vegetable Medley

2 small zucchini (about 5" long)
2 small onions (about 2" in diameter)
1 red bell pepper (5 ounces)
1/8 teaspoon onion powder
1/8 teaspoon garlic powder
1/8 teaspoon paprika
dash of ground black pepper
1/8 teaspoon salt (optional)

Prepare vegetables by cutting zucchini, onions, and peppers in large bite-size pieces. Sprinkle seasonings on vegetables and toss to coat evenly. Proceed with either method listed below.

BARBECUE: *Spray a sheet of aluminum foil about 12" × 12" with nonstick cooking spray. After spraying the foil, set it on the barbecue grill. Start the grill at this point. When the barbecue is hot, arrange vegetables on the foil. Close the hood and cook for 15 minutes, turning the vegetables with a spatula halfway through the cooking time.

STOVE TOP: Spray a large skillet or griddle with nonstick cooking spray. Place vegetables on the hot griddle and sprinkle with seasonings. Stir-fry about 10–15 minutes or until vegetables are tender.

Nonstick cooking spray is flammable. Do not spray near open flame or heated surfaces.

This is the best recipe for zucchini that I have tried, and it is also colorful. The outdoor grill gives these vegetables an excellent smoked flavor everyone will enjoy. This recipe can also be prepared in a skillet.

Makes 2 1/2 cups
4 servings

Each Serving
1/4 recipe

Carb Servings
1/2

Exchanges
1 vegetable

Nutrient Analysis
calories 29
total fat 0g
saturated fat 0mg
cholesterol 0mg
sodium 3mg
total carbohydrate 6g
dietary fiber 2g
sugars 3g
protein 1g

Makes 3 cups
6 servings

_____

Each Serving
1/2 cup

Carb Servings
0

Exchanges
1 vegetable

Nutrient Analysis
calories 27
total fat 0g
saturated fat 0mg
cholesterol 0mg
sodium 2mg
total carbohydrate 5g
dietary fiber 2g
sugars 2g
protein 1g

Green Bean Sauté

1 medium onion, chopped (1 cup)
1 cup sliced mushrooms
1 teaspoon minced garlic
1 can (14.5 ounces) cut green beans, drained*

Spray a skillet with nonstick cooking spray.

Sauté onions, mushrooms, and garlic. Add green beans and heat thoroughly.

Sodium is figured for no added salt.

Italian Green Beans

1 tablespoon dried chopped onion (or 1/3 cup sliced
green onion)
2 tablespoons water
1/2 medium green bell pepper, chopped
1 can (14.5 ounces) green beans, drained*
1 medium tomato, chopped
1/4 teaspoon dried basil
1/8 teaspoon dried rosemary

If using dried onion, soak in 2 tablespoons of water for a
few minutes.

Mix all ingredients in a microwave-safe bowl. Cover,
venting the lid, and cook on high in the microwave for 3
minutes, stirring halfway through cooking time, or until
green pepper is tender.

Sodium is figured for no added salt.

*This is a simple but
flavorful way to dress
up green beans.
You can easily substitute
stewed tomatoes (drained)
for fresh.*

Makes 3 cups
6 servings

Each Serving
1/2 cup

Carb Servings
0

Exchanges
1 vegetable

Nutrient Analysis
calories 26
total fat 0g
saturated fat 0mg
cholesterol 0mg
sodium 5mg
total carbohydrate 5g
dietary fiber 2g
sugars 2g
protein 1g

Take advantage of vegetables in season when making this recipe and substitute whatever is plentiful. Although the serving size is listed as one-half cup, you'll probably want seconds.

Makes 4 cups
8 servings

Each Serving
1/2 cup

Carb Servings
1/2

Exchanges
1 vegetable

Nutrient Analysis
calories 36
total fat 1g
saturated fat 0mg
cholesterol 1mg
sodium 34mg
total carbohydrate 6g
dietary fiber 1g
sugars 2g
protein 2g

Harvest Vegetable Stir-Fry

1/2 cup chopped onion
1 cup chopped green bell pepper
1 cup diced eggplant, not peeled
1 cup sliced zucchini
1 cup sliced yellow summer squash
1 cup chopped tomatoes
1 teaspoon Italian seasoning
1/4 teaspoon salt (optional)
2 tablespoons grated Parmesan cheese

Spray a large skillet with nonstick cooking spray. Add onion and bell pepper and stir-fry over medium-high heat for 2–3 minutes.

Stir in eggplant, zucchini, and yellow squash. Stir-fry for 4–5 minutes. Stir in tomatoes and seasonings. Heat thoroughly. Sprinkle with Parmesan cheese before serving.

Ranch-Style Vegetables

1 cup cauliflower, bite-sized pieces
1 cup broccoli florets
3/4 cup sliced carrots
1/2 cup sliced celery
1/3 cup chopped onion
1/4 teaspoon dried dill weed
1 1/2 tablespoons lemon juice
2 tablespoons fat-free or reduced-fat ranch-style dressing

Fill a 1 1/2 quart casserole or microwave-safe dish with vegetables. Add dill and lemon juice. Follow directions below for microwave or conventional oven.

MICROWAVE OVEN: Cover, venting the lid, and cook on high 5–8 minutes or until vegetables are done to your liking. Be sure to stir vegetables every 2 minutes. Drain. Mix in dressing.

CONVENTIONAL OVEN: Preheat oven to 350 degrees. Cover and bake 20–30 minutes until vegetables are done to your liking. Drain. Mix in dressing.

Any combination of fresh vegetables can be used in this dish, so keep this in mind when you're overloaded with garden vegetables.

Makes 2 cups
4 servings

Each Serving
1/2 cup

Carb Servings
1/2

Exchanges
2 vegetable

Nutrient Analysis
calories 49
total fat 0g
saturated fat 0mg
cholesterol 0mg
sodium 113mg
total carbohydrate 10g
dietary fiber 2g
sugars 4g
protein 2g

Salads

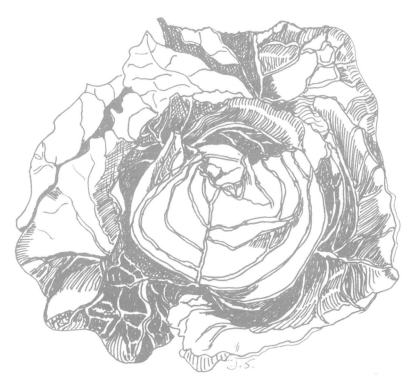

Side dish as well as main dish salads are included in this section. If some of your family members don't like cooked vegetables, serve salads and raw vegetables more often.

If you don't have the time or inclination to prepare lettuce and other fresh vegetables, be sure to check out the produce section in the grocery store for ready-to-use vegetables. It's a real time-saver!

Makes 8 cups
5 servings

Each Serving
about 1 1/2 cups

Carb Servings*
1

Exchanges*
1 fruit
1 vegetable
1/2 fat

Nutrient Analysis
calories 96
total fat 3g
saturated fat 0g
cholesterol 0mg
sodium 9mg
total carbohydrate 15g
dietary fiber 6g
sugars 10g
protein 3g

*Half of the grams of fiber have been subtracted from the grams of total carbohydrate when figuring Carb Servings and Exchanges.

Citrus Salad

1 grapefruit, peeled
1 orange, peeled
1 1/2 quarts of greens (12 ounces)
1 red onion, sliced thin (1 1/4 cups)
2 tablespoons cider vinegar
1 tablespoon lime juice
1 tablespoon canola oil
1 tablespoon water
1/4 teaspoon ground black pepper
1/4 teaspoon ground cumin
1/8 teaspoon salt (optional)

Cut fruit in bite-size pieces. Toss with lettuce and onion.

Mix remaining ingredients for dressing. Drizzle over salad and toss just before serving.

NOTE: One serving is an excellent source of fiber.

Frozen Fruit Salad

2 cans (8 ounces each) pineapple tidbits, in juice
1/4 cup granulated sugar or the equivalent in
    artificial sweetener
1 can (11 ounces) mandarin oranges, in juice, drained
1 package (8 ounces) frozen unsweetened
    strawberries, sliced
1 can (15 ounces) apricot halves, in juice, drained
2 bananas (7 inches each), sliced

Drain pineapple, reserving the liquid. Add water to the
pineapple juice to equal 1 cup and add sugar, stirring until
dissolved. Add the remaining ingredients to the juice.

Cover and freeze for several hours or overnight. Let sit
out about 30–45 minutes before serving.

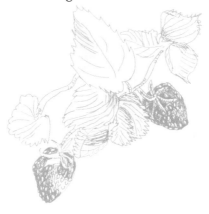

*This is a refreshing treat
on a hot summer day.
Serve this for lunch with
low-fat cottage cheese.*

Makes 6 cups
12 servings

Each Serving
1/2 cup

Carb Servings
1

Exchanges
1 fruit

Nutrient Analysis
calories 80
total fat 0g
saturated fat 0g
cholesterol 0mg
sodium 5mg
total carbohydrate 19g
dietary fiber 1g
sugars 13g
protein 1g

Makes 3 cups
6 servings

Each Serving
1/2 cup

Carb Servings
1

Exchanges
1 fruit

Nutrient Analysis
calories 57
total fat 0g
saturated fat 0g
cholesterol 0mg
sodium 36mg
total carbohydrate 13g
dietary fiber 1g
sugars 8g
protein 1g

Fruit Cocktail Salad

1 can (15.5 ounces) fruit cocktail, in juice
1 small package (0.3 ounces) sugar-free raspberry-flavored gelatin
1 cup applesauce, unsweetened

Drain fruit cocktail reserving the juice. Add water to the juice to equal 1 cup. Bring to a boil.

Dissolve gelatin in the boiling water/juice mixture. Add remaining ingredients. Chill until set.

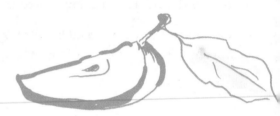

Mandarin Cottage Salad

2 cups low-fat cottage cheese

2 packages (0.3 ounces each) sugar-free orange-flavored gelatin

1 cup fat-free whipped topping

8 ounces vanilla fat-free yogurt, sweetened with artificial sweetener

1 can (11 ounces) mandarin oranges, in juice, drained

1 can (8 ounces) crushed pineapple, in juice, drained

Mix cottage cheese, gelatin, whipped topping, and yogurt in a medium bowl. Add fruit and mix well.

Cover and refrigerate until serving.

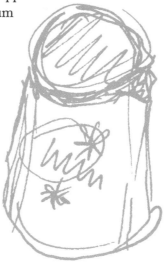

This light dish has a refreshing taste and a pretty pastel orange color.

Makes 5 cups
6 servings

Each Serving
about 3/4 cup

Carb Servings
1

Exchanges
1 fruit
2 lean meat

Nutrient Analysis
calories 128
total fat 1g
saturated fat 0g
cholesterol 5mg
sodium 432mg
total carbohydrate 15g
dietary fiber 0g
sugars 6g
protein 13g

Makes 3 cups
6 servings

Each Serving
1/2 cup

Carb Servings
1

Exchanges
1 fruit
1/2 fat

Nutrient Analysis
calories 73
total fat 3g
saturated fat 0g
cholesterol 0mg
sodium 70mg
total carbohydrate 12g
dietary fiber 1g
sugars 9g
protein 1g

Waldorf Salad

2 cups diced apples, unpeeled
2 teaspoons lemon juice
3 tablespoons light mayonnaise
2 tablespoons fat-free milk
1 cup diced celery
1/4 cup raisins

Toss apples with lemon juice in a medium bowl.

Mix mayonnaise and milk until smooth. Add remaining ingredients and mayonnaise mixture to apples. Toss to coat.

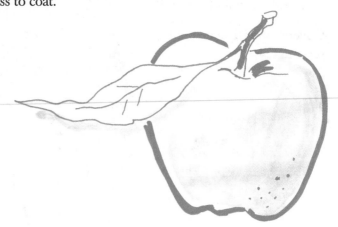

Broccoli and Raisin Salad

2 1/2 cups chopped fresh broccoli
1/2 cup raisins
1/4 cup sunflower seeds, unsalted
2 tablespoons diced red onion
2 tablespoons bacon-flavor soy bits
2 tablespoons fat-free plain yogurt
2 tablespoons light mayonnaise
1 1/2 tablespoons granulated sugar or the equivalent in artificial sweetener
1/2 tablespoon cider vinegar

Combine broccoli, raisins, sunflower seeds, onion, and soy bits.

Mix remaining ingredients together and add to broccoli mixture. Toss well to coat.

Chill 2 hours or longer for flavors to blend.

This is a family favorite and is a great dish to take to a potluck.

Makes 3 cups
6 servings

Each Serving
1/2 cup

Carb Servings
1

Exchanges
1 fruit
2 vegetable
1 fat

Nutrient Analysis
calories 132
total fat 5g
saturated fat 1g
cholesterol 0mg
sodium 103mg
total carbohydrate 18g
dietary fiber 2g
sugars 12g
protein 4g

*The vinegar adds a
special tang to this potato
salad.*

Makes 4 cups
8 servings

Each Serving
1/2 cup

Carb Servings
1

Exchanges
1 starch

Nutrient Analysis
calories 100
total fat 1g
saturated fat 0g
cholesterol 0mg
sodium 88mg
total carbohydrate 20g
dietary fiber 2g
sugars 3g
protein 3g

Hot German Potato Salad

1 pound potatoes, not peeled (about 4 cups, cubed)
3/4 cup chopped onion
1/2 teaspoon celery seeds
1/4 teaspoon salt (optional)
1/8 teaspoon ground black pepper
3/4 cup water
2 tablespoons unbleached all-purpose flour
1/3 cup cider vinegar
1 tablespoon granulated sugar or the equivalent in
    artificial sweetener
1/4 cup bacon-flavor soy bits

Scrub potatoes and cube. Place in medium saucepan and
cover with water. Bring to a boil. Cover, reduce heat, and
simmer 12 minutes or until potatoes are done. Drain.

Spray a skillet with nonstick cooking spray. Sauté onions
until done. Add celery seed, salt (optional), pepper, and
water. Simmer on low.

In a covered container, shake flour with vinegar to
prevent lumps. Add to onions and cook, stirring
constantly, until bubbly and thickened. Add sugar or
artificial sweetener and stir. Carefully stir in potatoes.
Serve hot, sprinkled with bacon bits.

Mozzarella and Tomato Salad

2 ounces reduced-fat mozzarella cheese, cut into very thin slices

2 medium tomatoes, cut into 1/4" slices

1 tablespoon red wine vinegar

1 teaspoon olive oil

1/2 teaspoon Dijon mustard

1/2 teaspoon dried parsley

1/4 teaspoon dried basil

1/4 teaspoon granulated sugar or the equivalent in artificial sweetener

1/8 teaspoon ground black pepper

Cut sliced cheese into pieces that are about half the size of the tomato slices.

On a large plate, alternate slices of tomato and mozzarella cheese. Arrange slices so that the top half of each tomato is not covered with cheese.

Mix remaining ingredients, and drizzle over salad, just before serving. Serve at room temperature.

Fresh tomatoes and deli-sliced mozzarella cheese make this a special dish. Have the tomatoes and cheese at room temperature for maximum flavor.

Makes 4 servings

Each Serving
1/4 recipe

Carb Servings
0

Exchanges
1 medium-fat meat

Nutrient Analysis
calories 72
total fat 4g
saturated fat 1g
cholesterol 8mg
sodium 90mg
total carbohydrate 5g
dietary fiber 1g
sugars 3g
protein 4g

Makes 4 cups
8 servings

Each Serving
1/2 cup

Carb Servings
1/2

Exchanges
1 vegetable
1/2 fat

Nutrient Analysis
calories 43
total fat 2g
saturated fat 0g
cholesterol 0mg
sodium 51mg
total carbohydrate 6g
dietary fiber 1g
sugars 4g
protein 1g

Summer Coleslaw

3 tablespoons light mayonnaise
3 tablespoons fat-free plain yogurt
2 teaspoons cider vinegar
1 tablespoon granulated sugar or the equivalent in artificial sweetener
1/4 teaspoon paprika
1/8 teaspoon ground black pepper
1/8 teaspoon salt (optional)
5 cups finely shredded cabbage (about 1 1/2 pounds)

Make the dressing by mixing the mayonnaise, yogurt, vinegar, sugar, paprika, pepper, and salt (optional).

Add to the cabbage and stir until well combined.

NOTE: For variety, add shredded carrots for color and add diced onion and diced green pepper for additional flavor.

Vegetable Pasta Salad

8 ounces rotini pasta, corkscrew shape (3 cups uncooked)
3/4 cup broccoli florets
3/4 cup cauliflower pieces
3/4 cup sliced cucumber, not peeled
3/4 cup sliced carrots
1/2 cup fat-free or reduced-fat Italian or
   ranch-style dressing

Cook pasta according to package directions, omitting salt and oil. Drain and cool.

Add vegetables and toss with dressing. Chill.

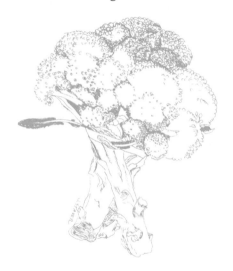

You can substitute your favorite fat-free or reduced-fat dressing in this recipe or use the one that we've listed. This recipe also works well with other vegetables such as zucchini and tomatoes.

Makes 7 cups
7 servings

___

Each Serving
1 cup

Carb Servings
2

Exchanges
1 1/2 starch
1 vegetable

Nutrient Analysis
calories 146
total fat 1g
saturated fat 0g
cholesterol 0mg
sodium 221mg
total carbohydrate 30g
dietary fiber 2g
sugars 3g
protein 5g

Makes 5 cups
5 servings

Each Serving
1 cup

Carb Servings
2

Exchanges
2 starch
  —with shrimp,
    2 starch, 2 lean meat

Nutrient Analysis
calories 132
  —with shrimp, 218
total fat 1g
  —with shrimp, 2g
saturated fat 0g
cholesterol 0mg
  —with shrimp, 177mg
sodium 186mg
  —with shrimp, 388mg
total carbohydrate 28g
dietary fiber 2g
sugars 3g
protein 3g
  —with shrimp, 22g

Confetti Salad

2 cups cooked brown rice (use quick-cooking)
1 1/3 cups frozen whole kernel corn
1/2 cup diced green bell pepper
1/2 cup diced red bell pepper
4 green onions, chopped
1 teaspoon dried thyme
1/3 cup fat-free or reduced-fat Italian dressing

Combine rice, vegetables, and seasoning.

Pour dressing over mixture and toss well.

VARIATION: *Confetti Shrimp Salad*–Add 1 pound cooked, cleaned, and deveined shrimp, and mix with vegetables before tossing with dressing.

Bean and Pasta Salad

8 ounces rotini noodles, corkscrew shape
   (3 cups uncooked)
1/2 cup chopped green onion
1 can (15 ounces) kidney beans, drained and rinsed
1 1/2 cups broccoli pieces
2 ounces (1/2 cup) grated reduced-fat cheddar cheese
6 tablespoons fat-free or reduced-fat Italian or
   ranch-style dressing
1 medium tomato, chopped

Cook noodles according to package directions, omitting salt and oil. Drain and cool.

In a large bowl, mix noodles, onion, kidney beans, broccoli, and cheese. Toss with the dressing.

Chill until serving. Toss with tomato just before serving.

NOTE: One serving is a good source of fiber.

Serve this as a side dish salad. You can substitute your favorite dressing.

Makes 8 cups
8 servings

Each Serving
1 cup

Carb Servings
2

Exchanges
2 starch
1 lean meat

Nutrient Analysis
calories 188
total fat 2g
saturated fat 1g
cholesterol 5mg
sodium 201mg
total carbohydrate 33g
dietary fiber 4g
sugars 2g
protein 9g

Makes 4 cups
8 servings

Each Serving
1/2 cup

Carb Servings
1

Exchanges
1 starch

Nutrient Analysis
calories 81
total fat 0g
saturated fat 0g
cholesterol 0mg
sodium 214mg
total carbohydrate 16g
dietary fiber 2g
sugars 2g
protein 4g

Black Bean Salad

1 can (15 ounces) black beans, drained and rinsed
1 1/3 cups frozen whole kernel corn
1 cup diced red bell pepper
4 green onions, chopped
1/4 teaspoon onion powder
1/4 teaspoon dried oregano
1/8 teaspoon garlic powder
1/8 teaspoon cayenne pepper
1/2 cup fat-free or reduced-fat Italian dressing

Combine all except the last ingredient. Pour dressing over mixture and toss well.

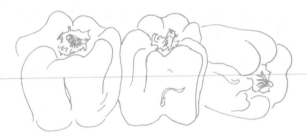

Beef, Bean, and Pasta Salad

6 ounces rotini noodles, corkscrew shape
(2 cups uncooked)
1/2 pound extra-lean ground beef or ground turkey (7% fat)
1/2 cup fat-free or reduced-fat ranch-style dressing
2–4 drops of Tabasco sauce
1/2 cup chopped green onion
1 can (15 ounces) kidney beans, drained and rinsed
4 ounces (1 cup) grated reduced-fat cheddar cheese
4 medium tomatoes, chopped

Cook noodles according to package directions, omitting salt and oil. Drain and cool.

Cook meat in a skillet that has been sprayed with nonstick cooking spray. Set aside.

Mix dressing and hot sauce. Add more Tabasco if you like a hot taste. Set aside.

In a large bowl, mix noodles, meat, onion, kidney beans, and cheese. Toss with the dressing. Chill until serving. Toss with tomatoes just before serving.

NOTE: One serving is an excellent source of fiber.

This is a great meal for a hot summer day. Keep this colorful dish in mind for potlucks.

Makes 9 cups
6 servings

Each Serving
1 1/2 cup

Carb Servings*
2 1/2

Exchanges*
2 1/2 starch
1 vegetable
2 lean meat

Nutrient Analysis
calories 294
total fat 7g
saturated fat 3g
cholesterol 45mg
sodium 400mg
total carbohydrate 43g
dietary fiber 6g
sugars 6g
protein 22g

*Half of the grams of fiber have been subtracted from the grams of total carbohydrate when figuring Carb Servings and Exchanges.

Served on a bed of baked tortilla chips, this salad is a family favorite. If you like things on the spicy side, add 2 drops of Tabasco to the dressing.

Makes 10 cups plus tortilla chips
5 servings

Each Serving
2 cups and 10 tortilla chips

Carb Servings**
2

Exchanges**
1 1/2 starch
2 vegetable
3 lean meat

Nutrient Analysis
calories 302
total fat 9g
saturated fat 3g
cholesterol 68mg
sodium 586mg
total carbohydrate 34g
dietary fiber 6g
sugars 3g
protein 23g

**Half of the grams of fiber have been subtracted from the grams of total carbohydrate when figuring Carb Servings and Exchanges.

Taco Salad

1/2 pound extra-lean ground beef or ground turkey (7% fat)
1/8 teaspoon chili powder
1/8 teaspoon garlic powder
1/8 teaspoon salt (optional)
1/2 head of lettuce, chopped (10 ounces)
1/2 cup chopped green onion
3 cups chopped tomato
1 can (15 ounces) kidney beans, drained and rinsed
4 ounces (1 cup) grated reduced-fat sharp cheddar cheese
3 ounces tortilla chips, baked type*
3/4 cup fat-free or reduced-fat thousand island or ranch-style dressing

Cook meat with the seasonings in a skillet that has been sprayed with nonstick cooking spray.

In a large bowl, mix lettuce, onion, tomatoes, kidney beans, cheese, and meat.

Divide tortilla chips on five individual plates and top with salad. Drizzle with dressing and serve immediately.

NOTE: One serving is an excellent source of fiber.

* Sodium is figured for salted. People on low-sodium diets should use unsalted baked tortilla chips.

Chicken Caesar Salad

1 pound skinless, boneless chicken breasts
1 1/2 quarts Romaine lettuce (12 ounces)
1/2 red onion, sliced thin
1/4 cup fat-free or reduced-fat Italian or Caesar dressing
4 teaspoons grated Parmesan cheese

Cook chicken breasts by one of the following methods:

MICROWAVE OVEN: Arrange in a microwave-safe baking dish in a circle on the outer portion of the dish. Cover, venting the lid, and microwave on high for 5 minutes, rearranging halfway through cooking time. Let set a few minutes before cutting into strips.

STOVE TOP: Place chicken in a pan and cover with water. Cover and simmer on low until tender (about 15–20 minutes). Drain liquid and save for soups. Cut chicken into strips.

Meanwhile, arrange salad greens on four plates. Arrange chicken and onion on salad greens. Drizzle 1 tablespoon of salad dressing over each salad. Sprinkle with Parmesan cheese.

For a hot summer evening, serve this simple salad with a whole-grain roll.

Makes 4 servings

Each Serving
1/4 recipe

Carb Servings
1/2

Exchanges
1 vegetable
3 lean meat

Nutrient Analysis
calories 168
total fat 4g
saturated fat 1g
cholesterol 71mg
sodium 286mg
total carbohydrate 6g
dietary fiber 2g
sugars 3g
protein 28g

Chicken Rainbow Salad

8 ounces tricolored rotini noodles, corkscrew shape
   (3 cups uncooked)
2 cups cooked, cubed chicken
1/2 medium cucumber, not peeled, sliced (1 cup)
1 cup sliced celery
1/2 red onion, sliced thin
1/2 cup light mayonnaise
1/4 cup fat-free sour cream
2 tablespoons fat-free milk
1 teaspoon dried dill weed
1 teaspoon salt (optional)
1/4 teaspoon ground black pepper

Cook pasta according to package directions, omitting salt and oil. Drain.

Meanwhile, in a large bowl, combine chicken, cucumber, celery, and onion. Mix in pasta.

In small bowl, blend mayonnaise, sour cream, milk, and seasonings. Toss dressing with salad mixture.

NOTE: One serving is a good source of fiber.

VARIATION: *Rainbow Vegetable Salad*—Omit chicken and reduce the mayonnaise to 1/3 cup. Serve as a side dish.

Hawaiian Chicken Salad

2 cups cooked and cubed chicken or turkey
2 cups cold cooked brown rice (use quick-cooking)
1 cup celery, diced
1 can (8 ounces) sliced water chestnuts, drained
2 cans (8 ounces each) pineapple tidbits, in juice, drained
1/3 cup light mayonnaise
2 tablespoons fat-free milk
1 tablespoon lemon juice
1/2 teaspoon salt (optional)
1/2 teaspoon curry powder
1/4 teaspoon ground black pepper

In a large bowl, mix chicken, rice, celery, water chestnuts, and pineapple.

In a smaller bowl, mix the remaining ingredients for the dressing.

Toss dressing with the chicken mixture.

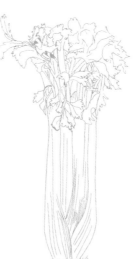

This delicious salad makes a tasty meal. It is a great recipe for using leftover turkey.

Makes 6 cups
4 servings

Each Serving
1 1/2 cups

Carb Servings
2

Exchanges
1 1/2 starch
1/2 fruit
3 lean meat

Nutrient Analysis
calories 294
total fat 9g
saturated fat 1g
cholesterol 59mg
sodium 209mg
total carbohydrate 28g
dietary fiber 2g
sugars 4g
protein 25g

Makes 5 cups
5 servings

Each Serving
1 cup

Carb Servings
1 1/2

Exchanges
1 starch
1 vegetable
2 lean meat

Nutrient Analysis
calories 169
total fat 2g
saturated fat 1g
cholesterol 29mg
sodium 151mg
total carbohydrate 22g
dietary fiber 2g
sugars 3g
protein 16g

Turkey Rotini Salad

4 ounces rotini noodles, corkscrew shape
  (1 1/2 cups uncooked)
3/4 cup broccoli florets
3/4 cup sliced carrots
1 1/2 cups cooked and cubed turkey breast
3 tablespoons fat-free or reduced-fat Italian or
  ranch-style dressing

Cook pasta according to package directions, omitting salt and oil. Drain and cool.

Add vegetables and turkey.
Toss with dressing.

Seafood Pasta Salad

4 ounces rotini noodles, corkscrew shape
  (1 1/2 cups uncooked)
8 ounces imitation crabmeat
4 ounces (1 cup) grated reduced-fat cheddar cheese
1 cup chopped celery
1/2 cup chopped red bell pepper
3–4 green onions, chopped
1/2 cup fat-free or reduced-fat ranch-style dressing

Prepare noodles according to package directions, omitting salt and oil. Drain and set aside.

In a large bowl, mix together crabmeat, cheese, celery, bell pepper, and onion. Toss with noodles and dressing.

Refrigerate to chill thoroughly before serving.

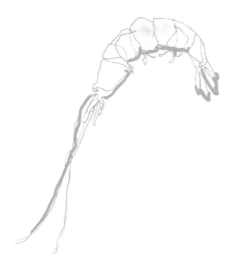

Here is a salad that is colorful, easy to prepare, and one that the whole family will enjoy. Either cooked shrimp or fresh crab can be used in place of imitation crab.

Makes 7 cups
7 servings

Each Serving
1 cup

Carb Servings
1

Exchanges
1 starch
2 lean meat

Nutrient Analysis
calories 159
total fat 4g
saturated fat 2g
cholesterol 28mg
sodium 384mg
total carbohydrate 19g
dietary fiber 1g
sugars 1g
protein 13g

Try this on a hot summer evening served on a bed of lettuce accompanied with sliced tomatoes.

Makes 6 cups
6 servings

Each Serving
1 cup

Carb Servings
1

Exchanges
1 starch
2 lean meat

Nutrient Analysis
calories 151
total fat 1g
saturated fat 0g
cholesterol 23mg
sodium 408mg
total carbohydrate 20g
dietary fiber 2g
sugars 2g
protein 16g

Tuna Macaroni Salad

4 ounces medium-size seashell pasta (2 cups uncooked)
1 cup chopped celery
1 cup chopped red bell pepper
4 green onions, sliced
2 cans (6 ounces each) water-packed tuna, drained
1/2 cup fat-free or reduced-fat ranch-style dressing

Cook macaroni according to package directions, omitting salt and oil. Drain.

Add and vegetables and tuna. Toss with dressing.

Refrigerate until serving.

Potatoes, Rice, Beans, and Pasta

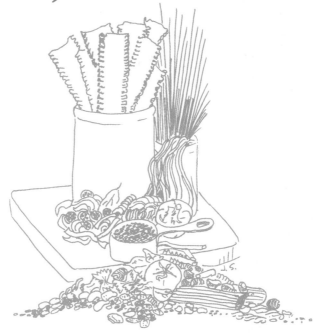

These side dishes will add variety to your meals. The bean dishes are favorites. A variety of pasta shapes are used throughout this book, but you can easily substitute with any pasta you have on hand.

These are a good substitute for traditional baked potatoes. Both yams and sweet potatoes have a slightly sweet taste. Yams have a bright orange pulp that gives more eye appeal than the sweet potatoes, which have a mustard-colored pulp. Sweet potatoes tend to take longer to cook than yams.

Makes 4 servings

Each Serving
1/2 sweet potato or yam

Carb Servings
1

Exchanges
1 starch

Nutrient Analysis
calories 60
total fat 0g
saturated fat 0g
cholesterol 0mg
sodium 6mg
total carbohydrate 14g
dietary fiber 2g
sugars 4g
protein 1g

Baked Sweet Potatoes or Yams

2 medium yams or sweet potatoes, not peeled

Scrub yams with a brush, and pierce skins with a fork. Proceed with oven or microwave method below.

CONVENTIONAL OVEN: Preheat oven to 400 degrees. Bake on a rack for 45–60 minutes or until soft when pierced with a fork.

MICROWAVE OVEN: Arrange in microwave at least 1" apart. Cook on high for 9–11 minutes. Turn potatoes and rotate 1/4 turn halfway through cooking time. Flesh should be soft when pierced with a fork. Let set for 5 minutes.

Barbecued Potatoes

1 pound small new potatoes, cut into quarters
  (about 4 cups), not peeled
1/8 teaspoon paprika
1/8 teaspoon ground black pepper
1/8 teaspoon salt (optional)

Spray a sheet of aluminum foil about 12" × 12" with nonstick cooking spray.* Set the foil on the barbecue. Start the grill.

Add potatoes to a microwave-safe casserole and sprinkle with seasonings. Cover, venting the lid, and microwave on high for 5 minutes, stirring after 1 1/2 minutes. Set aside.

When the barbecue is hot, arrange potatoes on the foil. Close hood and cook for 15 minutes, turning the potatoes halfway through cooking time.

NOTE: One serving is a good source of fiber.

Nonstick cooking spray is flammable. Do not spray near open flame or heated surfaces.

This a simple way to add variety to potatoes. By using the outdoor barbecue, your kitchen stays cool on a hot summer day. You can use baking potatoes instead of new potatoes, but be sure to cut into eighths. My favorite new potatoes are Yukon Gold. They have the best flavor.

Makes 4 servings

Each Serving
1/4 recipe

Carb Servings
2

Exchanges
2 starch

Nutrient Analysis
calories 126
total fat 0g
saturated fat 0g
cholesterol 0mg
sodium 9mg
total carbohydrate 29g
dietary fiber 3g
sugars 1g
protein 3g

Makes 2 cups
4 servings

Each Serving
1/2 cup

Carb Servings
2

Exchanges
2 starch

Nutrient Analysis
calories 136
total fat 0g
saturated fat 0g
cholesterol 0mg
sodium 17mg
total carbohydrate 31g
dietary fiber 3g
sugars 3g
protein 4g

Creamy Mashed Potatoes

3 medium potatoes, not peeled (about 1 pound)
1/4 cup fat-free sour cream
1/4 cup fat-free milk
1 tablespoon dried parsley
1 teaspoon dried dill weed (optional)
1/4 teaspoon salt (optional)
1/8 teaspoon ground black pepper

Scrub potatoes and cut into thick slices. Place in a medium saucepan, and cover with water. Bring to a boil. Reduce heat and simmer until potatoes are tender, about 15 minutes. Drain.

Mash potatoes, adding sour cream, milk, and seasonings. Continue to mash until no longer lumpy.

NOTE: One serving is a good source of fiber.

Oven-Fried Parmesan Potatoes

4 medium potatoes, not peeled (about 5 ounces each)
1 tablespoon canola oil
1 tablespoon grated Parmesan cheese
1/2 teaspoon garlic powder
1/2 teaspoon paprika
1/8 teaspoon ground black pepper
salt to taste (optional)

Preheat oven to 450 degrees. Scrub potatoes. Cut in wedges or strips.

Place potato slices in a plastic bag with the oil, and shake well to coat potatoes evenly.

Arrange potatoes, in a single layer, on a baking sheet that has been sprayed with nonstick cooking spray. Sprinkle with Parmesan cheese and seasonings. Bake for 30–35 minutes or until golden brown.

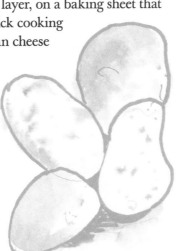

NOTE: One serving is a good source of fiber.

The addition of seasonings and cheese adds flavor and a golden color to these low-fat French fries.

Makes 5 servings

Each Serving
1/5 recipe

Carb Servings
2

Exchanges
2 starch

Nutrient Analysis
calories 159
total fat 3g
saturated fat 1g
cholesterol 1mg
sodium 32mg
total carbohydrate 29g
dietary fiber 3g
sugars 2g
protein 3g

This is a quick side dish that will dress up any meal.

Makes 3 cups
6 servings

Each Serving
1/2 cup

Carb Servings
2

Exchanges
2 starch
1/2 fat

Nutrient Analysis
calories 170
total fat 3g
saturated fat 1g
cholesterol 12mg
sodium 106mg
total carbohydrate 27g
dietary fiber 1g
sugars 4g
protein 9g

Creamy Dill Fettuccini

6 ounces uncooked fettuccini noodles
3 tablespoons unbleached all-purpose flour
1 1/2 cups fat-free milk, divided
2 teaspoons dried dill weed
1/4 teaspoon salt (optional)
1/8 teaspoon ground black pepper
2 ounces (1/2 cup) reduced-fat sharp cheddar cheese

Prepare noodles according to package instructions, omitting oil and salt. Drain and keep warm.

Meanwhile, prepare the sauce by combining the flour with 1/2 cup of milk in a covered container and shake well to prevent lumps. Pour into a 4-cup glass measuring cup along with the remainder of the milk and seasonings.

Cook in the microwave on high for 4–5 minutes, or until bubbly and thickened, stirring with a wire whisk every 60 seconds. Add cheese and stir until melted. Toss with noodles before serving.

Dijon Fettuccini

1/4 cup light mayonnaise
1/4 cup fat-free plain yogurt
2 teaspoons Dijon mustard
2 teaspoons dried parsley
2 teaspoons chopped garlic
6 ounces uncooked fettuccini noodles

Mix mayonnaise, yogurt, mustard, parsley, and garlic to make the sauce. Set aside.

Meanwhile, cook the fettuccini according to package directions, omitting oil and salt. Drain. Return to pan and add the sauce. Toss well. Cook on low until heated throughout.

These rich-tasting noodles are a good side dish with chicken, pork, seafood, or beef.

Makes 3 cups
6 servings

Each Serving
1/2 cup

Carb Servings
1 1/2

Exchanges
1 1/2 starch
1/2 fat

Nutrient Analysis
calories 144
total fat 4g
saturated fat 0g
cholesterol 0mg
sodium 117mg
total carbohydrate 24g
dietary fiber 1g
sugars 2g
protein 4g

This spicy-hot dish is a good accompaniment to any meat or seafood. You can make this into a complete meal by adding leftover poultry or meat.

Makes 6 cups
8 servings

Each Serving
3/4 cup

Carb Servings
1 1/2

Exchanges
1 1/2 starch
1/2 fat

Nutrient Analysis
calories 145
total fat 3g
saturated fat 0g
cholesterol 0mg
sodium 111mg
total carbohydrate 23g
dietary fiber 2g
sugars 2g
protein 6g

Szechuan Pasta

8 ounces egg noodles, "no yolk" type (4 cups uncooked)
2 cups sliced vegetables
  (green bell pepper, broccoli, pea pods, etc.)
1/2 cup fat-free chicken broth*
1 1/2 teaspoons cornstarch
1–2 tablespoons Szechuan sauce**
1/4 cup dry-roasted peanuts, unsalted

Prepare noodles according to package directions, omitting salt and oil. Drain and keep warm.

Spray a large skillet with nonstick cooking spray. Stir-fry vegetables until almost tender.

In a covered container, shake chicken broth and cornstarch to prevent lumps. Add to skillet with vegetables. Cook until bubbly and thickened, stirring constantly.

Add Szechuan sauce, peanuts, and noodles. Mix well.

Sodium is figured for reduced sodium.

**Found in the Asian section of the grocery store.*

Seasoned Black Beans

1 can (15 ounces) black beans, drained and rinsed
1/4 teaspoon onion powder
1/4 teaspoon dried oregano
1/8 teaspoon cayenne pepper
1/8 teaspoon garlic powder

Mix all ingredients in a microwave-safe dish. Cover, venting the lid, and microwave on high about 1–2 minutes, stirring halfway through cooking time.

NOTE: One serving is a good source of fiber.

Most canned black beans are not seasoned and need a little perking up before serving. This recipe makes a good side dish.

Makes 3 servings
1 cup

Each Serving
1/3 cup

Carb Servings
1

Exchanges
1 starch

Nutrient Analysis
calories 103
total fat 0g
saturated fat 0g
cholesterol 0mg
sodium 87mg
total carbohydrate 18g
dietary fiber 3g
sugars 1g
protein 7g

Any color of peppers works well in this recipe, but the red peppers are especially attractive. A combination of red, green, and yellow peppers can be used to create an eye-catching display.

Makes 6 halves
6 servings

Each Serving
1 pepper half

Carb Servings
2

Exchanges
1 1/2 starch
1 vegetable

Nutrient Analysis
calories 160
total fat 3g
saturated fat 1g
cholesterol 7mg
sodium 129mg
total carbohydrate 26g
dietary fiber 4g
sugars 3g
protein 9g

Black Bean Stuffed Peppers

3 bell peppers (about 6 ounces each)
1 can (15 ounces) black beans, drained and rinsed
3/4 cup frozen whole kernel corn
1 cup cooked quick-cooking brown rice
2 green onions, chopped
1 teaspoon ground cumin
1 teaspoon garlic powder
1/4 teaspoon salt (optional)
1/8 teaspoon cayenne pepper
2 ounces (1/2 cup) grated reduced-fat cheddar cheese

Preheat oven to 350 degrees. Pour 1/4 cup water in a 9" × 13" pan that has been sprayed with nonstick cooking spray. Set aside. Cut peppers in half lengthwise and remove seeds and membranes.

In a large bowl, combine remaining ingredients except cheese. Fill each pepper half with bean mixture. Arrange stuffed peppers, filling side up, in the pan. Cover with aluminum foil and bake for 30 minutes.

Sprinkle with cheese and return to oven, uncovered, for 5 minutes until cheese is melted. For smaller portions, cut each pepper half in half with a serrated knife before serving.

NOTE: One serving is a good source of fiber.

Spanish Rice and Beans

1 cup quick-cooking brown rice, uncooked
1/8 teaspoon ground cumin
1 1/4 cups fat-free chicken broth*
1 can (15 ounces) kidney beans, drained and rinsed
1 can (4 ounces) diced green chiles

Cook rice according to package directions, adding the cumin, substituting chicken broth for water, and omitting the salt.

When done, mix in remaining ingredients, and cover to heat thoroughly.

Sodium is figured for reduced sodium.

This is a colorful side dish that tastes great with Spanish Chicken, found on page 120. For a different flavor, try substituting black beans for the kidney beans.

Makes 4 cups
8 servings

Each Serving
1/2 cup

Carb Servings
1

Exchanges
1 starch

Nutrient Analysis
calories 85
total fat 1g
saturated fat 0g
cholesterol 0mg
sodium 20mg
total carbohydrate 16g
dietary fiber 2g
sugars 1g
protein 4g

Serve this recipe as a side dish with Mexican food. The green pepper and tomato add color as well as vitamins and minerals to this dish.

Makes 5 cups
5 servings

Each Serving
1 cup

Carb Servings
2

Exchanges
1 1/2 starch
1 vegetable

Nutrient Analysis
calories 131
total fat 1g
saturated fat 0g
cholesterol 0mg
sodium 89mg
total carbohydrate 27g
dietary fiber 1g
sugars 3g
protein 3g

Spicy Spanish Rice

1/3 cup salsa, thick and chunky
1 cup water
3/4 cup finely diced bell pepper
1 can (14.5 ounces) diced tomatoes, not drained*
1 1/2 cups quick-cooking brown rice, uncooked
1/4 teaspoon dried thyme
1/4 teaspoon salt (optional)
1/8 teaspoon ground black pepper

Spray a large skillet with nonstick cooking spray. Add all ingredients, and mix well. Bring to a boil. Reduce heat to low.

Cover and simmer 25 minutes or until most of the liquid is absorbed, stirring occasionally.

Sodium is figured for no added salt.

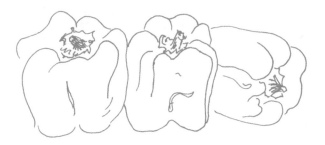

Zucchini Garden Casserole

3 cups sliced zucchini
2 cups chopped tomato
1/2 cup chopped red bell pepper
1/2 cup chopped green bell pepper
1/4 cup fat-free Italian dressing
1 cup quick-cooking brown rice, uncooked
1 tablespoon grated Parmesan cheese (optional)

Spray a 2-quart microwave-safe casserole with nonstick cooking spray. Add vegetables and dressing. Cover, venting the lid, and microwave on high for 10 minutes, stirring after every 3 minutes.

Meanwhile, cook rice according to package directions, omitting salt. Spoon the vegetables and juice over rice when serving. Sprinkle with Parmesan cheese (optional).

NOTE: One serving is a good source of fiber.

The addition of Italian dressing adds a zing to this dish.

Makes 4 cups of vegetables and 2 cups of rice
4 servings

Each Serving
1 cup of vegetables and
  1/2 cup of rice

Carb Servings
2

Exchanges
1 starch
2 vegetable

Nutrient Analysis
calories 149
total fat 1g
saturated fat 0g
cholesterol 0mg
sodium 200mg
total carbohydrate 30g
dietary fiber 3g
sugars 7g
protein 5g

Sandwiches

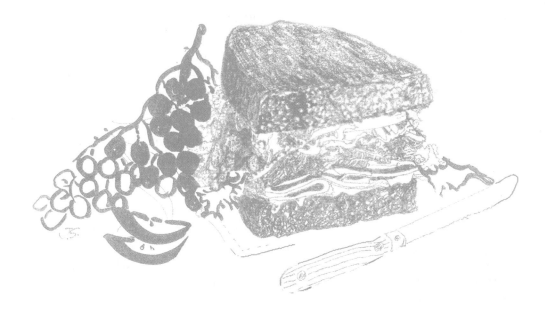

Using different breads and fillings adds variety to traditional sandwiches. The recipes that use several vegetables are particularly tasty.

This recipe may be used as part of a meal, or the quesadillas can be cut into wedges for an appetizer. The microwave makes this especially quick.

Makes 4 servings

Each Serving
1/4 recipe

Carb Servings
2 1/2

Exchanges
2 1/2 starch
1 lean meat

Nutrient Analysis
calories 250
total fat 4g
saturated fat 1g
cholesterol 10mg
sodium 409mg
total carbohydrate 38g
dietary fiber 3g
sugars 3g
protein 15g

Black Bean Quesadillas

1 can (15 ounces) black beans, drained and rinsed
2 tablespoons salsa, thick and chunky
1/4 teaspoon onion powder
1/4 teaspoon dried oregano
1/8 teaspoon cayenne pepper
1/8 teaspoon garlic powder
2 tablespoons chopped green onion
4 whole-wheat tortillas (8 inch)
2 ounces (1/2 cup) grated reduced-fat mozzarella cheese

Mash beans. Add salsa, seasonings, and onion. Mix well.

Microwave oven: Spoon filling onto half of each tortilla. Top with cheese and fold each tortilla in half. Microwave on high for 60 seconds, rotating 1/4 turn halfway through cooking time.

Skillet or griddle: Divide filling onto 2 tortillas. Top with cheese and the remaining 2 tortillas. Spray griddle or skillet with nonstick cooking spray, and brown quesadillas on both sides. Cut in half or quarters before serving.

NOTE: One serving is a good source of fiber.

Cheese and Chile Quesadillas

1/4 cup diced green chiles
4 whole-wheat tortillas (8 inch)
2 ounces (1/2 cup) grated reduced-fat mozzarella cheese

MICROWAVE OVEN: Divide chiles onto half of each tortilla. Top with cheese, and fold each tortilla in half. Microwave on high for 60 seconds, rotating 1/4 turn halfway through cooking time.

SKILLET OR GRIDDLE: Divide chiles onto 2 tortillas. Top with cheese and the remaining 2 tortillas. Spray griddle or skillet with nonstick cooking spray, and brown quesadillas on both sides. Cut in half or quarters before serving.

Serve these for a light meal when you really don't think you have time to make dinner. Add fresh sliced fruit for a side dish. These also make a good appetizer.

Makes 4 servings

Each Serving
1/4 recipe

Carb Servings
1 1/2

Exchanges
1 1/2 starch
1 lean meat

Nutrient Analysis
calories 173
total fat 3g
saturated fat 1g
cholesterol 8mg
sodium 310mg
total carbohydrate 25g
dietary fiber 1g
sugars 3g
protein 9g

Makes 4 servings

Each Serving
1/4 recipe

Carb Servings
1 1/2

Exchanges
1 1/2 starch
2 lean meat

Nutrient Analysis
calories 229
total fat 6g
saturated fat 2g
cholesterol 23mg
sodium 479mg
total carbohydrate 24g
dietary fiber 1g
sugars 3g
protein 20g

Tuna Quesadillas

1 can (6 ounces) water-packed tuna, drained
1 tablespoon light mayonnaise or salad dressing
4 whole-wheat tortillas (8 inch)
2 ounces (1/2 cup) grated reduced-fat sharp
   cheddar cheese

Flake tuna with a fork. Combine with mayonnaise.

MICROWAVE OVEN: Spoon filling onto half of each tortilla. Top with cheese and fold each tortilla in half. Microwave on high for 60 seconds, rotating 1/4 turn halfway through cooking time.

SKILLET OR GRIDDLE: Divide filling onto 2 tortillas. Top with cheese and the remaining 2 tortillas. Spray griddle or skillet with nonstick cooking spray, and brown quesadillas on both sides. Cut in half or quarters before serving.

Broiled Seafood Muffins

2 tablespoons light salad dressing or mayonnaise
4 ounces cooked shrimp, crab, or fish
2 whole-grain English muffins, split
1 ounce (1/4 cup) grated reduced-fat sharp
   cheddar cheese

Mix seafood with salad dressing.

Toast muffins. Top with
seafood and cheese. Broil until
cheese melts.

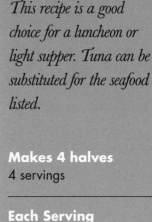

*This recipe is a good
choice for a luncheon or
light supper. Tuna can be
substituted for the seafood
listed.*

Makes 4 halves
4 servings

Each Serving
1 half

Carb Servings
1

Exchanges
1 starch
1 lean meat

Nutrient Analysis
calories 136
total fat 4g
saturated fat 1g
cholesterol 62mg
sodium 378mg
total carbohydrate 14g
dietary fiber 2g
sugars 3g
protein 10g

Makes 6 slices
6 servings

Each Serving
1 slice

Carb Servings
2

Exchanges
1 1/2 starch
1 vegetable
2 medium-fat meat

Nutrient Analysis
calories 200
total fat 4g
saturated fat 1g
cholesterol 10mg
sodium 410mg
total carbohydrate 31g
dietary fiber 2g
sugars 6g
protein 9g

Ricotta Pizza

1 (10 ounces) thin pizza crust
1/2 cup pizza sauce
1 cup reduced-fat ricotta cheese
1 cup thinly sliced green bell pepper
1 cup thinly sliced onion
1 cup thinly sliced tomato

Preheat oven to 450 degrees. Place pizza crust on pizza pan and spread pizza sauce over surface.

Spread ricotta cheese over sauce and top with peppers and onions.

Bake for 8–10 minutes. Arrange tomato slices over pizza.

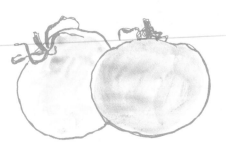

Beef and Cabbage Sandwich

1/2 pound top sirloin steak, cut into bite-size pieces
3/4 cup sliced onion
2 cups shredded cabbage
1/8 teaspoon salt (optional)
dash ground black pepper
1 teaspoon caraway seeds
1 teaspoon dried parsley
2 whole-wheat pita breads (2 ounces each)
1/2 cup fat-free plain yogurt
2 teaspoons Dijon mustard

Spray a skillet with nonstick cooking spray. Brown the steak and onion. Add cabbage, salt (optional), pepper, caraway, and parsley. Continue to stir-fry until vegetables are tender and beef is cooked to your liking.

Cut pita bread in half and microwave on high for 20 seconds or until warm.

Meanwhile, mix yogurt with mustard. Spread 2 tablespoons of yogurt mixture in each pita bread half. Fill with beef stir-fry.

This is a great pocket sandwich. Try this recipe on one of those hurried evenings.

Makes 4 half sandwiches
4 servings

Each Serving
1 half sandwich

Carb Servings
1

Exchanges
1 starch
2 lean meat

Nutrient Analysis
calories 180
total fat 3g
saturated fat 1g
cholesterol 33mg
sodium 220mg
total carbohydrate 19g
dietary fiber 1g
sugars 4g
protein 16g

Makes 4 half sandwiches
4 servings

Each Serving
1 half sandwich

Carb Servings
1

Exchanges
1 starch
2 lean meat

Nutrient Analysis
calories 147
total fat 2g
saturated fat 0g
cholesterol 30mg
sodium 144mg
total carbohydrate 15g
dietary fiber 1g
sugars 3g
protein 16g

Chicken Stir-Fry Sandwich

1/2 pound skinless, boneless chicken breasts, cut into strips
3/4 cup sliced red bell pepper
3/4 cup sliced green bell pepper
1/4 cup chopped green onion
1 teaspoon chopped garlic
1 teaspoon dried parsley
1/4 teaspoon dried thyme
1/8 teaspoon salt (optional)
1/16 teaspoon ground black pepper
2 whole-wheat pita breads, 2 ounces each
1/4 cup fat-free plain yogurt or ranch-style dressing

Spray a skillet with nonstick cooking spray. Add chicken, vegetables, and seasonings. Stir-fry until chicken is done and vegetables are to your liking.

Cut pita bread in half and microwave on high for 20 seconds or until warm.

Spread 1 tablespoon of yogurt or dressing in each pita bread half. Fill with chicken stir-fry.

Turkey Reuben Sandwich

1 cup sauerkraut
8 slices of whole-grain bread
8 ounces sliced lean turkey
2 ounces (1/2 cup) grated reduced-fat Swiss cheese

Preheat to 400 degrees. Drain and rinse sauerkraut. Rinse and drain again. Squeeze out moisture.

Toast bread. On each of 4 slices, place 2 ounces turkey, 1/4 cup sauerkraut, and 1/4 of the Swiss cheese. Top with remaining slices of bread. Wrap in aluminum foil and bake for 10 minutes or until thoroughly heated and cheese is melted.

NOTE: One serving is an excellent source of fiber.

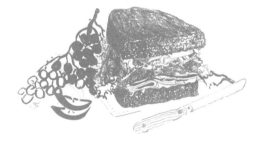

This is a low-fat version of a high-fat sandwich. Use of lower-fat ingredients and the elimination of butter makes this tasty and yet low-fat. Rinsing the sauerkraut helps to reduce the sodium, but it does not eliminate it.

Makes 4 sandwiches
4 servings

Each Serving
1 sandwich

Carb Servings
2

Exchanges
2 starch
3 lean meat

Nutrient Analysis
calories 272
total fat 6g
saturated fat 2g
cholesterol 56mg
sodium 570mg
total carbohydrate 28g
dietary fiber 5g
sugars 11g
protein 26g

Makes 2 half sandwiches
1 serving

Each Serving
2 halves

Carb Servings
2

Exchanges
2 starch
1 vegetable
1 lean meat

Nutrient Analysis
calories 221
total fat 1g
saturated fat 0g
cholesterol 4mg
sodium 637mg
total carbohydrate 35g
dietary fiber 4g
sugars 6g
protein 15g

Garden Deli Sandwich

1 whole-wheat pita bread, 2 ounces
1/4 cup fat-free cream cheese
1/2 cup sliced cucumber, not peeled
4 tomato slices
1 cup chopped lettuce

Cut pita bread in half. Spread cream cheese inside pita bread. Add sliced vegetables and lettuce.

NOTE: One serving is a good source of fiber.

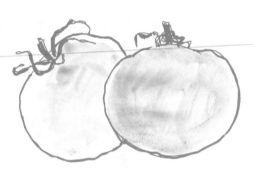

Vegetable Stir-Fry Sandwich

1 cup sliced zucchini
1 1/2 cups sliced red pepper
1 1/4 cups sliced onion
1/2 teaspoon dried parsley
1/8 teaspoon dried thyme
1/8 teaspoon salt (optional)
dash ground black pepper
2 whole-wheat pita breads, 2 ounces each
1/2 cup fat-free cream cheese

Spray a skillet with nonstick cooking spray. Add vegetables and seasonings. Stir-fry until vegetables are cooked to your liking.

Cut pita bread in half and microwave on high for 20 seconds or until warm. Spread 2 tablespoons of cream cheese in each pita bread half. Fill with stir-fried vegetables.

This sandwich is a good choice for a luncheon or a light supper. Feel free to vary the vegetables to whatever is in season.

Makes 4 half sandwiches
4 servings

Each Serving
1 half sandwich

Carb Servings
1

Exchanges
1 starch
1 vegetable
1 lean meat

Nutrient Analysis
calories 129
total fat 1g
saturated fat 0g
cholesterol 1mg
sodium 278mg
total carbohydrate 20g
dietary fiber 2g
sugars 2g
protein 8g

Meatless

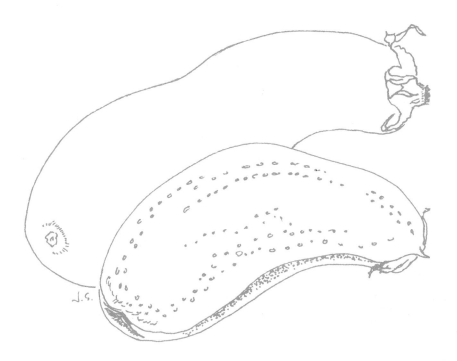

You don't have to be a vegetarian to appreciate the good-tasting recipes in this section. My family's favorites are the Eggplant Parmesan and the Rice and Bean Burritos. Both are easy enough for kids to prepare.

This is a great choice for a brunch or luncheon. Serve with a fruit cup or orange wedges.

Makes 8 servings

Each Serving
1/8 recipe

Carb Servings
1

Exchanges
1/2 starch
1 vegetable
2 lean meat

Nutrient Analysis
calories 134
total fat 3g
saturated fat 1g
cholesterol 10mg
sodium 291mg
total carbohydrate 13g
dietary fiber 1g
sugars 3g
protein 13g

Broccoli Quiche

3 whole-wheat tortillas (8-inch)
2 cups broccoli pieces
1/2 cup sliced green onion
4 ounces (1 cup) grated reduced-fat cheddar cheese
2 cups egg substitute (equal to 8 eggs)
1/4 cup fat-free milk
1/4 teaspoon paprika
8 tomato slices

Preheat oven to 350 degrees. Spray a 9" pie pan with nonstick cooking spray. Cut 2 tortillas in half and place each half in the pan so that the rounded edge is 1/4 inch above the rim. Place the remaining tortilla in the center of the pan.

Add broccoli, onion, and cheese. Mix eggs with milk, and pour over top. Sprinkle with paprika.

Bake for 45 minutes or until a sharp knife inserted in the center comes out clean. Let sit for 10 minutes before cutting into 8 wedges. Top each piece with a tomato slice.

Vegetarian Sausage Quiche

3 whole-wheat tortillas (8-inch)
8 vegetarian sausage links
2 ounces (1/2 cup) grated reduced-fat cheddar cheese
1 can (6.5 ounces) sliced mushrooms, drained and rinsed
2 1/2 cups egg substitute (equal to 10 eggs)
1/2 cup fat-free milk
1/2 tablespoon dried parsley
1/4 teaspoon paprika

Preheat oven to 350 degrees. Spray a 9" pie pan with nonstick cooking spray. Cut 2 tortillas in half and place each half in the pan so that the rounded edge is 1/4 inch above the rim. Place the remaining tortilla in the center of the pan.

Place the sausage links over the tortillas in a spoke-like fashion. Top with cheese and mushrooms. Mix eggs with milk and pour over top. Sprinkle with parsley and paprika.

Bake for 45–50 minutes or until a sharp knife inserted in the center comes out clean. Let sit for 10 minutes before cutting into 8 wedges.

This appealing dish is assembled in minutes. It's great for a brunch or breakfast served with fresh fruit.

Makes 8 servings

Each Serving
1/8 recipe

Carb Servings
1

Exchanges
1 starch
2 lean meat

Nutrient Analysis
calories 157
total fat 4g
saturated fat 1g
cholesterol 5mg
sodium 463mg
total carbohydrate 14g
dietary fiber 1g
sugars 2g
protein 16g

This is an easy supper or brunch dish that will be a favorite for anyone who likes Mexican food. Seasoned Black Beans on page 165 can be substituted for the refried beans. Serve with salsa.

Makes 8 servings

Each Serving
1/8 recipe

Carb Servings
1 1/2

Exchanges
1 1/2 starch
2 lean meat

Nutrient Analysis
calories 180
total fat 4g
saturated fat 1g
cholesterol 10mg
sodium 485mg
total carbohydrate 21g
dietary fiber 2g
sugars 2g
protein 15g

Spanish Quiche

3 whole-wheat tortillas (8-inch)
1 can (16 ounces) fat-free refried beans
1 can (4 ounces) diced green chiles
1/2 cup sliced green onion
4 ounces (1 cup) grated reduced-fat cheddar cheese
1 3/4 cups egg substitute (equal to 7 eggs)
1/4 cup fat-free milk
1/4 teaspoon paprika

Preheat oven to 350 degrees. Spray a 9" pie pan with nonstick cooking spray. Cut 2 tortillas in half and place each half in the pan so that the rounded edge is 1/4 inch above the rim. Place the remaining tortilla in the center of the pan.

Spread beans over tortillas. Top with chiles, onion, and cheese. Mix eggs with milk and pour over top. Sprinkle with paprika.

Bake for 50 minutes or until a sharp knife inserted in the center comes out clean. Let sit for 10 minutes before cutting into 8 wedges.

Cheese and Tortilla Lasagna

1 can (14.5 ounces) diced tomatoes, not drained*
1 can (8 ounces) tomato sauce*
2/3 cup frozen whole kernel corn
1 can (4 ounces) diced green chiles
1 teaspoon chili powder
3/4 teaspoon ground cumin
1/4 teaspoon ground black pepper
1/8 teaspoon garlic powder
1/16 teaspoon cayenne pepper
1/4 cup egg substitute (equal to 1 egg)
2 cups low-fat cottage cheese
7 corn tortillas, cut into strips
2 ounces (1/2 cup) grated reduced-fat cheddar cheese

Preheat oven to 350 degrees. Mix canned tomatoes with tomato sauce, corn, chiles, and seasonings. Set aside. Mix egg substitute with cottage cheese and set aside.

Spray an 8" × 8" pan with nonstick cooking spray. Layer in this order: 1/3 tortillas, 1/3 cheese mixture, 1/3 tomato mixture, and repeat twice, ending with tomato mixture.

Bake for 30 minutes or until bubbly. Sprinkle with grated cheese and return to oven until melted.

Sodium is figured for no added salt.

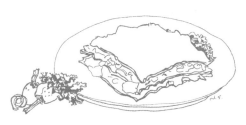

The crunch of the corn adds an interesting texture to this dish. If you are serving a crowd, double this recipe and cook in a 9" × 13" pan.

Makes 6 servings

Each Serving
1/6 recipe

Carb Servings
2

Exchanges
1 1/2 starch
1 vegetable
2 lean meat

Nutrient Analysis
calories 220
total fat 4g
saturated fat 2g
cholesterol 10mg
sodium 515mg
total carbohydrate 29g
dietary fiber 2g
sugars 3g
protein 18g

This is a healthy variation of macaroni and cheese that your family will enjoy. *Macaroni and Sausage Casserole,* in the "Ground Meat and Sausage" section, is a variation of this recipe.

Makes 8 cups
5 servings

Each Serving
1 1/2 cups

Carb Servings
3

Exchanges
2 1/2 starch
1 vegetable
2 lean meat

Nutrient Analysis
calories 298
total fat 6g
saturated fat 1g
cholesterol 17mg
sodium 238mg
total carbohydrate 43g
dietary fiber 3g
sugars 6g
protein 17g

Macaroni and Cheese Casserole

8 ounces elbow macaroni (2 cups uncooked)
4 cups broccoli pieces
1 1/2 cups fat-free milk, divided
3 tablespoons unbleached all-purpose flour
1/4 teaspoon salt (optional)
1/8 teaspoon ground black pepper
4 ounces (1 cup) grated reduced-fat sharp
   cheddar cheese

Prepare macaroni according to package directions, omitting salt and oil. Drain and keep warm.

Meanwhile, add broccoli to a 2-quart microwave-safe casserole dish. Cover, venting the lid, and cook in the microwave on high for 4 minutes, mixing halfway through cooking time. Keep warm.

Combine 1/2 cup milk with flour in covered container and shake well to prevent lumps. Pour flour mixture and the rest of the milk into a 4-cup glass measuring cup, and cook in the microwave on high for 4–5 minutes, stirring after each minute with a wire whisk until bubbly and thickened. Mix in seasonings and cheddar cheese.

Add cooked noodles and sauce to the broccoli. Mix well.

NOTE: One serving is a good source of fiber.

Eggplant Lasagna

1 cup low-fat ricotta cheese
1 cup low-fat cottage cheese
2 tablespoons dried parsley
1 teaspoon chopped garlic
1 small eggplant (about 14 ounces), not peeled
5 cups spaghetti sauce (less than 4 grams of fat
   per 4 ounces)
12 ounces lasagna noodles, uncooked
4 ounces (1 cup) grated reduced-fat mozzarella cheese
1/4 cup grated Parmesan cheese

Preheat oven to 350 degrees. Mix ricotta cheese, cottage
cheese, parsley, and garlic. Slice eggplant about 1/4 inch
thick.

In a 9" × 13" pan that has been sprayed with nonstick
cooking spray, pour in 1 cup spaghetti sauce. Arrange
1/3 of the noodles in the pan so that they touch but do
not overlap.

Layer in this order: half the eggplant, mozzarella cheese,
1 cup spaghetti sauce, 1/3 lasagna noodles, cheese
mixture, remainder of the eggplant, 1 cup spaghetti sauce,
the remainder of the lasagna noodles, and the remainder
of the spaghetti sauce. Sprinkle with Parmesan cheese.
Bake, covered tightly with aluminum foil, for 1 hour.

NOTE: One serving is a good source of fiber.

   This recipe is higher in sodium and should be
   limited by those on a low-sodium diet.

*You save time with this
recipe because you don't
precook the noodles. This
is another meatless meal
that your whole family will
enjoy. You can substitute
1 1/2 cups of fresh
sliced vegetables, such as
zucchini, for each layer of
eggplant.*

Makes 10 servings

Each Serving
1/10 recipe

Carb Servings
3

Exchanges
2 starch
2 vegetable
1 lean meat

Nutrient Analysis
calories 270
total fat 5g
saturated fat 2g
cholesterol 10mg
sodium 701mg
total carbohydrate 41g
dietary fiber 3g
sugars 9g
protein 16g

Quick, easy, and delicious! This dish is so quick to put together that you will make it often.

Makes 4 servings

Each Serving
1/4 recipe

Carb Servings
1 1/2

Exchanges
1 starch
2 vegetable
1 medium-fat meat

Nutrient Analysis
calories 188
total fat 5g
saturated fat 3g
cholesterol 16mg
sodium 623mg
total carbohydrate 24g
dietary fiber 3g
sugars 10g
protein 11g

Eggplant Parmesan

2 1/2 cups spaghetti sauce (less than 4 grams of fat per 4 ounces)
1 medium eggplant, not peeled (about 1 1/2–2 pounds)
4 ounces (1 cup) grated reduced-fat mozzarella cheese
grated Parmesan cheese (optional)

Preheat oven to 350 degrees. Spray a 9" × 13" pan with nonstick cooking spray. Pour 1/2 cup of sauce in pan.

Slice eggplant 1/2" thick. Arrange half of the slices in the baking pan. Top with 1 cup of sauce, half of the mozzarella cheese, the remainder of the eggplant slices, and the remainder of the sauce.

Cover with aluminum foil and bake for 45–55 minutes. Top with the remainder of the mozzarella cheese and return to oven, uncovered, until cheese is melted. Serve with Parmesan cheese (optional).

NOTE: One serving is a good source of fiber.

Harvest Primavera

8 ounces egg noodles, "no yolk" type (4 cups uncooked)
1 cup chopped onion
1 cup sliced zucchini
1 cup sliced yellow summer squash
1 cup chopped bell pepper, red, green, or yellow
2 cups spaghetti sauce (less than 4 grams of fat
   per 4 ounces)
1 tablespoon grated Parmesan cheese

Cook noodles according to package directions, omitting salt and oil. Drain and keep warm. Proceed with either stove top or microwave directions below.

STOVE TOP: Mix vegetables and spaghetti sauce in a saucepan and simmer until vegetables are tender, about 20–30 minutes. Spoon vegetable mixture over noodles and serve with Parmesan cheese.

MICROWAVE OVEN: Mix vegetables and spaghetti sauce in a microwave-safe 2-quart casserole. Cover, venting the lid, and cook on high for 8 minutes, stirring halfway through cooking time. Spoon vegetable mixture over noodles and serve with Parmesan cheese.

NOTE: One serving is a good source of fiber.

This recipe takes advantage of fresh vegetables in season.

Makes 4 cups of noodles and 4 cups of sauce
5 servings

Each Serving
3/4 cup of noodles and
   3/4 cup of sauce

Carb Servings
3

Exchanges
2 1/2 starch
2 vegetable

Nutrient Analysis
calories 241
total fat 2g
saturated fat 0g
cholesterol 1mg
sodium 341mg
total carbohydrate 47g
dietary fiber 4g
sugars 11g
protein 9g

Italian Curry Pasta

The addition of curry with fresh tomatoes makes this dish uniquely flavorful. If you are not especially fond of curry, use the lesser amount, and you will still like this recipe.

Makes 5 cups
4 servings

Each Serving
1 1/4 cups

Carb Servings
3

Exchanges
2 1/2 starch
2 vegetable

Nutrient Analysis
calories 260
total fat 3g
saturated fat 1g
cholesterol 3mg
sodium 89mg
total carbohydrate 49g
dietary fiber 5g
sugars 10g
protein 10g

5 cups chopped tomatoes
1 cup chopped onion
1 teaspoon chopped garlic
1 teaspoon ground cumin
1 or 2 teaspoons curry powder
1/2 teaspoon dried cilantro
1/2 teaspoon salt (optional)
6 ounces angel hair pasta, uncooked
2 tablespoons grated Parmesan cheese

Spray a skillet with nonstick cooking spray. Add vegetables and seasonings. Cook for 15–20 minutes or until thickened.

Meanwhile, prepare pasta according to package directions, omitting salt and oil. Drain.

Pour sauce over pasta and toss. Serve sprinkled with Parmesan cheese.

NOTE: One serving is an excellent source of fiber.

Pesto Linguini

12 ounces linguini, uncooked
1/4 cup pesto sauce
grated Parmesan cheese (optional)

Prepare linguini according to package directions, omitting salt and oil. Drain. Return to pan and toss with pesto sauce. Serve with Parmesan cheese.

It doesn't get much easier than this. Serve as a main dish or as a side dish. When using pesto sauce, limit the amount you use because it is high in fat, and just a small amount provides a good flavor.

Makes 6 cups
6 servings

Each Serving
1 cup

Carb Servings
3

Exchanges
3 starch
1 fat

Nutrient Analysis
calories 253
total fat 6g
saturated fat 1g
cholesterol 2mg
sodium 76mg
total carbohydrate 42g
dietary fiber 1g
sugars 2g
protein 8g

Makes 4 cups filling and 8 tortillas
8 servings

Each Serving
1/2 cup filling and
  1 tortilla

Carb Servings
2 1/2

Exchanges
2 starch
1 vegetable
1 lean meat

Nutrient Analysis
calories 215
total fat 2g
saturated fat 1g
cholesterol 0mg
sodium 258mg
total carbohydrate 40g
dietary fiber 3g
sugars 2g
protein 9g

Rice and Bean Burritos

2 tablespoons salsa, thick and chunky
1/3 cup water
1 green bell pepper, finely diced (1 cup)
1 can (14.5 ounces) diced tomatoes, not drained*
3/4 cup quick-cooking brown rice, uncooked
1/4 teaspoon dried thyme
1/4 teaspoon salt (optional)
1/8 teaspoon ground black pepper
1 can (15 ounces) black beans, drained and rinsed
8 whole-wheat tortillas (8-inch)
fat-free sour cream (optional)
salsa, thick and chunky (optional)

Spray a large skillet with nonstick cooking spray. Add salsa, water, bell pepper, tomatoes, rice, and seasonings. Bring to a boil. Reduce heat to low. Cover and simmer 15 minutes. Stir in drained beans. Continue to cook on low, covered, for 10 minutes or until most of the liquid is absorbed, stirring occasionally.

Warm tortillas in microwave oven on high, in a covered microwave-safe container, for 1 minute, rotating 1/4 turn halfway through cooking time. Or, heat in the oven, wrapped in aluminum foil, for 10 minutes at 350 degrees.

Serve 1/2 cup filling in each tortilla. Top with optional fat-free sour cream and/or salsa before folding.

NOTE: One serving is a good source of fiber.

Sodium is figured for no added salt.

Vegetable Lasagna

Béchamel Sauce:

2 cups fat-free milk, divided
2 tablespoons unbleached all-purpose flour
2 ounces (1/2 cup) grated reduced-fat mozzarella cheese
1/2 cup grated Parmesan cheese
1/8 teaspoon dried oregano
1/8 teaspoon ground nutmeg

4 cups spaghetti sauce (less than 4 grams of fat per 4 ounces)
1 small eggplant (about 12 ounces), not peeled, sliced thin
12 ounces lasagna noodles, uncooked
1 1/2 cups thinly sliced fresh vegetables such as broccoli, carrots, and zucchini
1 package (10 ounces) frozen spinach, thawed, drained, and squeezed

Prepare Béchamel sauce: Pour 1/2 cup of milk in a covered container. Add flour and shake well to prevent lumps. In a 4-cup glass measuring cup, combine flour mixture with remaining milk. Cook on high in the microwave for 5–6 minutes (stirring well with a wire whisk after each minute) or until bubbly. Add the remaining sauce ingredients. Set aside.

Preheat oven to 350 degrees. In a 9" × 13" pan that has been sprayed with nonstick cooking spray, pour in 1/3 spaghetti sauce and layer in this order: eggplant, 1/3 lasagna noodles, 1/3 spaghetti sauce, fresh vegetables, 1/3 lasagna noodles, Béchamel sauce, spinach, the remainder of the lasagna noodles, and the remainder of the spaghetti sauce.

Cover tightly with aluminum foil and bake for 1 hour.

NOTE: One serving is a good source of fiber.

You save time with this recipe because you don't precook the noodles. It is very attractive and a great way to use fresh garden vegetables.

Makes 10 servings

Each Serving
1/10 recipe

Carb Servings
3

Exchanges
2 starch
2 vegetable
1 lean meat

Nutrient Analysis
calories 247
total fat 4g
saturated fat 2g
cholesterol 8mg
sodium 475mg
total carbohydrate 41g
dietary fiber 3g
sugars 11g
protein 12g

 MEATLESS | **195**

Poultry

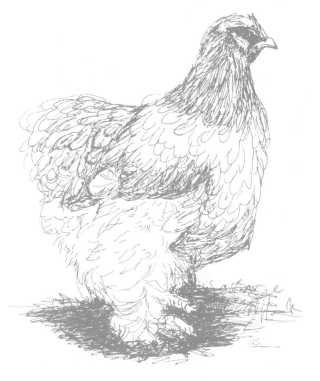

The variety of recipes in this section offers more ways to prepare lean poultry. Be sure to keep skinless, boneless chicken breasts in your freezer so you can prepare a meal on very short notice. You'll find additional poultry recipes in the sections "Sandwiches," "Soups and Stews," and "Salads."

This is a quick meal that goes well with Citrus Salad on page 136. Kidney beans or pinto beans can be substituted for the black beans.

Makes 6 servings

Each Serving
3/4 cup mixture and
   1 tortilla

Carb Servings
2 1/2

Exchanges
2 starch
1 vegetable
2 lean meat

Nutrient Analysis
calories 255
total fat 3g
saturated fat 1g
cholesterol 23mg
sodium 354mg
total carbohydrate 40g
dietary fiber 3g
sugars 5g
protein 18g

Chicken and Black Bean Burritos

1/2 pound skinless, boneless chicken breasts, cut into
   bite-size pieces
1 teaspoon ground cumin
1 teaspoon garlic powder
1 can (15 ounces) black beans, drained and rinsed
3/4 cup frozen whole kernel corn
1/2 cup salsa, thick and chunky
1 1/2 cups diced green bell pepper
6 whole-wheat tortillas (8 inch)
fat-free sour cream (optional)
salsa, thick and chunky (optional)

Brown chicken in a skillet that has been sprayed with nonstick cooking spray. Add all but the tortillas and optional ingredients. Continue to cook until the chicken and vegetables are done.

Heat tortillas in a covered microwave-safe container in the microwave for 1 minute, rotating 1/4 turn halfway through cooking.

To serve, spoon 3/4 cup of chicken mixture onto a tortilla. Fold ends in and roll up burrito style. Serve as is or with salsa and fat-free sour cream.

NOTE: One serving is a good source of fiber.

Chicken and Red Pepper Burritos

1/2 pound skinless, boneless chicken breasts, cut into
  bite-size pieces
3/4 cup chopped red bell pepper
2 tablespoons chopped onion
1 teaspoon chopped garlic
1/2 teaspoon dried cilantro
1/2 teaspoon dried basil
1/4 teaspoon ground cumin
1/2 cup diced tomato
2 ounces (1/2 cup) grated reduced-fat cheddar cheese
5 whole-wheat tortillas (8 inch)

Preheat oven to 350 degrees. Spray skillet with nonstick
cooking spray. Over medium heat, sauté chicken, bell
pepper, onion, garlic, and seasonings until chicken is
cooked. Mix in tomatoes and cheese.

Spoon filling onto each tortilla. Roll tightly, and place
seam side down in 8" × 8" baking dish that has been
sprayed with nonstick cooking spray.

Bake 15 minutes or until heated through.

This is a simple dish that will be enjoyed by the entire family.

Makes 5 servings

Each Serving
1 filled tortilla

Carb Servings
2

Exchanges
1 1/2 starch
1 vegetable
2 lean meat

Nutrient Analysis
calories 226
total fat 5g
saturated fat 1g
cholesterol 36mg
sodium 315mg
total carbohydrate 27g
dietary fiber 1g
sugars 4g
protein 19g

Use leftover chicken or turkey in this simple dish. Serve over hot biscuits, toast, noodles, or rice.

Makes 3 cups
4 servings

Each Serving
3/4 cup

Carb Servings
1

Exchanges
1 starch
3 lean meat

Nutrient Analysis
calories 214
total fat 4g
saturated fat 1g
cholesterol 60mg
sodium 198mg
total carbohydrate 26g
dietary fiber 2g
sugars 4g
protein 29g

Chicken à la King

3 tablespoons unbleached all-purpose flour
1 1/2 cups fat-free milk, divided
1 1/2 teaspoons instant chicken bouillon*
2 cups cooked and cubed chicken or turkey
1 cup frozen peas
1 jar (2 ounces) pimento, drained
1/8 teaspoon ground black pepper

Combine flour with 1/2 cup cold milk in covered container and shake well to prevent lumps. Follow directions below for stove top or microwave oven.

STOVE TOP: Pour into a saucepan along with the rest of the milk and the chicken bouillon. Bring to a boil, stirring constantly until bubbly and thickened. Lower heat and add remaining ingredients. Continue cooking until peas and chicken are heated.

MICROWAVE OVEN: Pour into a 2-quart microwave-safe casserole along with the rest of the milk and the chicken bouillon. Cook on high for 4–5 minutes, stirring after each minute with a wire whisk, until mixture is bubbly and thickens. Add remaining ingredients. Cover, venting the lid, and continue to cook on high for 2–3 minutes or until peas and chicken are heated throughout.

*Sodium is figured for salt-free.

Chicken Chop Suey

1 pound skinless, boneless chicken breasts, cut into strips
   (or 2 cups cooked, cubed chicken or turkey)
2 cups sliced celery
1 cup sliced onion
1 cup fat-free chicken broth*
1 tablespoon lite soy sauce
1/4 teaspoon salt (optional)
2 1/2 tablespoons cornstarch
1/4 teaspoon ginger
1 tablespoon molasses
1/4 cup water
1 can (16 ounces) bean sprouts, drained
   (or 1 1/2 cups fresh)

Spray a large frying pan with nonstick cooking spray, and
brown chicken. If using cooked meat, there is no need
to brown. Add celery, onion, broth, soy sauce, and salt
(optional). Cover and simmer for 5–10 minutes.

Meanwhile, mix cornstarch, ginger, molasses, and water.
Stir into hot mixture and cook until thickened. Add bean
sprouts and heat thoroughly. Serve over noodles or quick-
cooking brown rice.

Sodium is figured for reduced sodium.

This is an easy dish that tastes great over noodles or rice. You can substitute leftover turkey, which makes this a good choice after Thanksgiving.

Makes 5 cups
4 servings

Each Serving
1 1/4 cups

Carb Servings
1

Exchanges
3 vegetable
3 lean meat

Nutrient Analysis
calories 197
total fat 3g
saturated fat 1g
cholesterol 68mg
sodium 361mg
total carbohydrate 15g
dietary fiber 2g
sugars 2g
protein 27g

Chicken Curry

This spicy dish will appeal to anyone who likes curry. Use the lesser amount of curry if you do not like spicy dishes.

Makes 4 cups curry and 2 cups rice
4 servings

Each Serving
1 cup curry and
   1/2 cup rice

Carb Servings
2 1/2

Exchanges
2 starch
1 vegetable
3 lean meat

Nutrient Analysis
calories 278
total fat 4g
saturated fat 1g
cholesterol 52mg
sodium 189mg
total carbohydrate 37g
dietary fiber 4g
sugars 7g
protein 24g

3/4 pound skinless, boneless chicken breasts,
   cut into strips
3/4 cup chopped onion
1 tablespoon chopped garlic
1–2 tablespoons curry powder
1 1/2 cups diced apple, not peeled
1/4 teaspoon salt (optional)
1 1/2 cups fat-free chicken broth, divided*
2 tablespoons unbleached all-purpose flour
2 cups cooked quick-cooking brown rice

Spray skillet with nonstick cooking spray. Stir-fry chicken with onion and garlic until chicken is browned. Add curry, apple, salt (optional), and 1 cup of broth. Cover and simmer for 10 minutes or until chicken is done.

In a covered container, shake flour with 1/2 cup of broth to prevent lumps. Stir into chicken mixture and bring to a boil, stirring constantly until thickened. Serve over cooked rice.

NOTE: One serving is a good source of fiber.

Sodium is figured for reduced sodium.

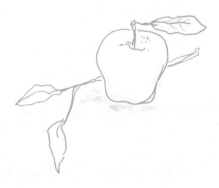

Chicken Fricassee

1 pound skinless, boneless chicken breasts, cut into strips
1 cup sliced onions
1 cup sliced mushrooms
1 1/2 cups sliced bell pepper (red or green)
1 1/2 cups fat-free chicken broth*
1 teaspoon lemon juice
1/2 teaspoon dried thyme
1/4 teaspoon salt (optional)
1/2 cup fat-free milk
4 tablespoons unbleached all-purpose flour
3 tablespoons sherry or fat-free chicken broth

Spray skillet with nonstick cooking spray. Over medium heat, stir-fry chicken with onions, mushrooms, and bell pepper until chicken is lightly browned. Add all but the last three ingredients. Cover and simmer for 10 minutes.

Meanwhile, in a covered container, shake milk with flour to prevent lumps. Stir into chicken along with the sherry. Bring to a boil, stirring constantly until thickened.

Sodium is figured for reduced sodium.

The sherry adds a special flavor to this popular dish. However, chicken broth can be substituted for the sherry. Serve over rice, mashed potatoes, or noodles.

Makes 4 cups
4 servings

Each Serving
1 cup

Carb Servings
1

Exchanges
1/2 starch
1 vegetable
3 lean meat

Nutrient Analysis
calories 216
total fat 3g
saturated fat 1g
cholesterol 70mg
sodium 218mg
total carbohydrate 14g
dietary fiber 2g
sugars 4g
protein 30g

This is an attractive and simple dish. Beef or pork can be substituted for the chicken.

Makes 6 cups
4 servings

Each Serving
1 1/2 cups

Carb Servings
2 1/2

Exchanges
2 starch
2 vegetable
3 lean meat

Nutrient Analysis
calories 315
　—with beef, 321
total fat 4g
　—with beef, 6g
saturated fat 1g
　—with beef, 2g
cholesterol 69mg
　—with beef, 64mg
sodium 96mg
　—with beef, 84mg
total carbohydrate 38g
dietary fiber 4g
sugars 11g
protein 32g
　—with beef, 29g

Chicken Hungarian Goulash

4 1/2 ounces ziti pasta, tube shape
　(1 1/2 cups uncooked)
1 pound skinless, boneless chicken breasts, cut into
　bite-size pieces
3/4 cup chopped onion
1 1/2 cups chopped green bell pepper
1 can (14.5 ounces) diced tomatoes, not drained*
1 can (8 ounces) tomato sauce*
1/2–1 tablespoon paprika
1 tablespoon dried parsley
1/2 teaspoon salt (optional)
1/8 teaspoon ground black pepper

Cook noodles according to package directions, omitting salt and oil. Drain and set aside.

Meanwhile, spray a large skillet with nonstick cooking spray. Add chicken, onion, and green pepper and stir-fry until browned. Add remaining ingredients, including noodles, and simmer until chicken is cooked.

NOTE: One serving is a good source of fiber.

* *Sodium is figured for no added salt.*

VARIATION: *Beef Hungarian Goulash*–Substitute 1 pound top sirloin for the chicken.

Chicken Medley

1 pound skinless, boneless chicken breasts, cut into strips
3 cups (6 ounces) fresh snow pea pods
2 cups sliced celery
1 1/2 cups sliced red bell pepper
1/2 cup sliced onion
2 cups fat-free chicken broth*
1 tablespoon lite soy sauce
1/4 teaspoon ground ginger
1/4 teaspoon salt (optional)
3 tablespoons cornstarch
1/2 cup water

Brown chicken in a large skillet that has been sprayed with nonstick cooking spray. Add all but the last two ingredients and simmer, covered, until chicken is cooked, about 10 minutes.

Meanwhile, mix cornstarch with water. Stir into hot mixture and simmer, stirring constantly, until thickened. Serve over rice or noodles.

NOTE: One serving is a good source of fiber.

Sodium is figured for reduced sodium.

This is a colorful dish that can be varied by using different vegetables and meats. It's great served over rice or noodles.

Makes 6 cups
4 servings

Each Serving
1 1/2 cups

Carb Servings
1

Exchanges
1/2 starch
2 vegetable
3 lean meat

Nutrient Analysis
calories 207
total fat 3g
saturated fat 1g
cholesterol 69mg
sodium 438mg
total carbohydrate 16g
dietary fiber 3g
sugars 4g
protein 29g

Ramen Chicken

This is a complete meal in a pot. Substitute other vegetables for variety. It has an excellent taste and also looks appealing.

Makes 7 cups
4 servings

Each Serving
1 3/4 cups

Carb Servings
2 1/2

Exchanges
2 starch
1 vegetable
3 lean meat

Nutrient Analysis
calories 318
total fat 4g
saturated fat 1g
cholesterol 69mg
sodium 498mg
total carbohydrate 37g
dietary fiber 3g
sugars 5g
protein 34g

1 pound skinless, boneless chicken breasts, cut into bite-size pieces
2 3/4 cups fat-free chicken broth*
1 tablespoon lite soy sauce
1 teaspoon ground ginger
1/8 teaspoon ground black pepper
1/4 teaspoon salt (optional)
1/2 teaspoon garlic powder
1 1/2 cups sliced onion
1 cup sliced mushrooms
1/2 cup sliced carrots
3 cups (6 ounces) fresh snow pea pods
4 ounces coil vermicelli (fine noodles), uncooked
1 tablespoon cornstarch
1/4 cup water

Spray a large skillet with nonstick cooking spray and brown chicken. Add all but the last three ingredients and bring to a boil. Add noodles. Reduce heat to low, cover, and simmer for 8–10 minutes or until vegetables are almost done.

Mix cornstarch with water. Add to skillet. Bring to a boil, stirring until thickened.

NOTE: One serving is a good source of fiber.

Sodium is figured for reduced sodium.

Skillet Chicken with Tomatoes

1 pound skinless, boneless chicken breasts, cut into bite-size pieces
1 1/4 cups onion, thinly sliced
1 carrot, sliced
1 celery stalk, sliced
2 teaspoons chopped garlic
1 teaspoon dried oregano
1/2 teaspoon dried parsley
1/4 teaspoon salt (optional)
1 can (14.5 ounces) stewed tomatoes, not drained*
1 1/2 cups fat-free chicken broth*
2 cups sliced potatoes, not peeled

Spray a large skillet with nonstick cooking spray. Sauté chicken until browned.

Add remaining ingredients to skillet and simmer over medium heat until potatoes are tender.

NOTE: One serving is a good source of fiber.

Sodium is figured for no added salt/reduced sodium.

This is a flavorful and easy top-of-the-stove dish that is a complete meal.

Makes 6 cups
4 servings

Each Serving
1 1/2 cups

Carb Servings
2

Exchanges
1 starch
2 vegetable
3 lean meat

Nutrient Analysis
calories 255
total fat 3g
saturated fat 1g
cholesterol 66mg
sodium 296mg
total carbohydrate 29g
dietary fiber 4g
sugars 7g
protein 28g

Serve this great-tasting Chinese dish with rice or low-fat Ramen noodles. If you like spicy-hot dishes, use the larger amount of Szechuan sauce.

Makes 6 cups
4 servings

Each Serving
1 1/2 cups

Carb Servings
1/2

Exchanges
2 vegetable
4 lean meat

Nutrient Analysis
calories 232
total fat 9g
saturated fat 2g
cholesterol 69mg
sodium 414mg
total carbohydrate 9g
dietary fiber 3g
sugars 4g
protein 30g

Szechuan Chicken

1 pound skinless, boneless chicken breasts, cut into bite-size pieces
1/4 cup teriyaki sauce
2 teaspoons chopped garlic
1 1/2 cups sliced red bell pepper
1 1/2 cups sliced green bell pepper
16 green onions, cut into 1-inch pieces
2–4 tablespoons Szechuan sauce
1/3 cup dry-roasted peanuts, unsalted

Combine chicken with teriyaki sauce and marinate at least 1 hour in the refrigerator. Drain and discard marinade.

Spray a large skillet with nonstick cooking spray, and brown chicken with garlic.

Add remaining ingredients except peanuts and stir-fry for 1–2 minutes or until vegetables are tender and chicken is cooked. Add peanuts.

NOTE: One serving is a good source of fiber.

Black Bean and Chicken Casserole

1 pound skinless, boneless chicken breasts, cut into strips
1/4 teaspoon each: chili powder and salt (optional)
1/8 teaspoon ground black pepper
1 cup quick-cooking brown rice, uncooked
1 1/4 cups fat-free chicken broth*
1 can (15 ounces) black beans, drained and rinsed
1 can (4 ounces) diced green chiles
1/8 teaspoon each: ground cumin, cayenne pepper, and garlic powder
1/4 teaspoon each: onion powder and dried oregano
2 ounces (1/2 cup) grated reduced-fat cheddar cheese

Spray a 9" × 13" baking pan or microwave-safe dish with nonstick cooking spray. Arrange chicken in pan and top with chili powder, salt (optional), and pepper. Follow directions below for conventional oven or microwave.

CONVENTIONAL OVEN: Preheat oven to 350 degrees. Bake for 20 minutes or until chicken is done.

MICROWAVE OVEN: Cover, venting the lid, and cook on high for 6–8 minutes, depending on thickness of chicken. Rotate dish halfway through cooking time.

Meanwhile, cook rice according to package directions, substituting chicken broth for water and omitting salt. When rice is done, mix in black beans, chiles, and remaining seasonings. Pour drippings from cooked chicken into rice mixture and mix well. Spread over chicken. Top with grated cheese. Return to conventional oven for 5 minutes (microwave oven for 30 seconds) or until cheese is melted.

NOTE: One serving is a good source of fiber.

Sodium is figured for reduced sodium.

This dish has excellent flavor. Kidney beans can be substituted for black beans.

Makes about 6 cups
5 servings

Each Serving
1 1/4 cups

Carb Servings
2

Exchanges
1 1/2 starch
1 vegetable
3 lean meat

Nutrient Analysis
calories 252
total fat 4g
saturated fat 1g
cholesterol 59mg
sodium 359mg
total carbohydrate 26g
dietary fiber 4g
sugars 1g
protein 30g

The addition of rice and vegetables makes this one-dish meal great-tasting and colorful. Asparagus or Brussels sprouts can be used in place of the broccoli for variety.

Makes 5 servings

Each Serving
1/5 recipe

Carb Servings
2

Exchanges
1 1/2 starch
1 vegetable
3 lean meat

Nutrient Analysis
calories 302
total fat 6g
saturated fat 3g
cholesterol 69mg
sodium 276mg
total carbohydrate 27g
dietary fiber 3g
sugars 5g
protein 34g

Chicken and Broccoli in Cheese Sauce

1 cup quick-cooking brown rice, uncooked
1/2 cup finely chopped onion
1/2 cup finely chopped celery
1 tablespoon dried parsley
1 teaspoon instant chicken bouillon*
1/4 teaspoon dried thyme
1 cup of boiling water
1 pound skinless, boneless chicken breasts, cut into strips
4 cups broccoli spears

Cheese Sauce
1 1/2 cups fat-free milk, divided
3 tablespoons unbleached all-purpose flour
1/4 teaspoon salt (optional)
1/8 teaspoon ground black pepper
3 ounces reduced-fat sharp cheddar cheese,
   cut into small pieces

Preheat oven to 450 degrees. Spray a 9" × 13" baking pan with nonstick cooking spray. Add rice, onion, celery, parsley, bouillon, thyme, and water, stirring to mix well. Top with chicken breasts and broccoli spears. Cover with aluminum foil and bake for 30 minutes, or until chicken is no longer pink.

Meanwhile, prepare cheese sauce. Combine 1/2 cup milk with flour in covered container and shake well to prevent lumps. Pour into a 4-cup glass measuring cup along with the rest of the milk and seasonings. Cook in the microwave on high for 4–5 minutes, stirring with a wire whisk every 60 seconds until mixture is bubbly and thickens. Mix in the cheese and stir until melted. Pour sauce over broccoli and chicken before serving.

NOTE: One serving is a good source of fiber.

Sodium is figured for salt-free.

Chicken and Stuffing Casserole

1 cup chopped onion
1 cup chopped celery
2 1/2 cups fat-free chicken broth,* divided
6 cups (6 ounces) packaged unseasoned stuffing mix (cubes)
1/2 teaspoon dried thyme
1/2 teaspoon dried sage
1/8 teaspoon dried marjoram
1 pound skinless, boneless chicken breasts, cut into strips
2 tablespoons unbleached all-purpose flour
1 tablespoon dried parsley

Preheat oven to 350 degrees. In a medium saucepan, combine onion, celery, and 1 1/2 cups broth. Simmer, covered, on low until vegetables are soft. Add stuffing and seasonings. Mix well until blended. Spread in an 8" × 8" pan that has been sprayed with nonstick cooking spray. Top with chicken strips.

Meanwhile, in a covered container, combine 1 cup chicken broth with flour and shake well to prevent lumps. Pour into a 4-cup glass measuring cup and cook in the microwave on high for 3–4 minutes, stirring with a wire whisk after each minute until mixture is bubbly and thickens. Pour over chicken breasts. Sprinkle with parsley. Cover and bake for 30 minutes or until chicken is no longer pink.

NOTE: If you use leftover cooked turkey, reduce the cooking time to 20 minutes or until all ingredients are thoroughly heated.

Sodium is figured for reduced sodium.

This is a family favorite. You can easily substitute leftover turkey for the chicken.

Makes 6 servings

Each Serving
1/6 recipe

Carb Servings
2

Exchanges
1 1/2 starch
1 vegetable
2 lean meat

Nutrient Analysis
calories 230
total fat 3g
saturated fat 1g
cholesterol 46mg
sodium 341mg
total carbohydrate 27g
dietary fiber 1g
sugars 2g
protein 23g

Makes 8 cups
5 servings

Each Serving
about 1 1/2 cups

Carb Servings
2 1/2

Exchanges
2 1/2 starch
2 lean meat

Nutrient Analysis
calories 285
total fat 3g
saturated fat 1g
cholesterol 55mg
sodium 136mg
total carbohydrate 37g
dietary fiber 2g
sugars 2g
protein 27g

Chicken Noodle Casserole

8 ounces rotini noodles, corkscrew shape
  (3 cups uncooked)
1 pound skinless, boneless chicken breasts, cut into
  bite-size pieces
1/2 cup chopped celery
1/2 cup chopped onion
1 cup fat-free chicken broth*
1 jar (2 ounces) pimento, drained
2 tablespoons dried parsley
1/2 teaspoon garlic powder
1/2 teaspoon dried thyme
1/2 teaspoon salt (optional)
1/8 teaspoon ground black pepper

Prepare noodles according to package directions, omitting salt and oil. Drain and set aside.

In a large skillet that has been sprayed with nonstick cooking spray, brown chicken with celery and onion. Add the remaining ingredients and simmer on low until meat is tender and vegetables are cooked. Mix in noodles and continue to simmer on low until half of the liquid is absorbed. Remove from heat, cover, and let sit for 5 minutes before serving.

NOTE: One cup of sliced mushrooms can be added and sautéed with the celery and onion.

Sodium is figured for reduced sodium.

Patio Chicken and Rice

2 tablespoons cornstarch
1/4 cup water
1/2 cup fat-free milk
2 cups fat-free chicken broth*, divided
1/2 teaspoon ground black pepper
1/4 teaspoon salt (optional)
1/3 cup dried chopped onion
1 1/2 cups quick-cooking brown rice, uncooked
1 can (13 ounces) sliced mushrooms, drained and rinsed
1 jar (2 ounces) pimento, drained
8–10 skinless chicken parts (thighs, legs, and
   breast quarters)
10 small (4") carrots, scrubbed
1/2 teaspoon paprika

Preheat oven to 350 degrees. In a 4-cup glass measuring cup, mix cornstarch with water. Add milk and 1 cup of chicken broth. Heat on high in microwave for 4–5 minutes, stirring every 60 seconds until bubbly and thickened. Add the pepper, salt, and onion. Set aside.

Spread rice in a 4-quart covered casserole that has been sprayed with nonstick cooking spray. Pour 1 cup of broth over rice. Top with mushrooms, pimento, chicken, and carrots. Pour cornstarch mixture over all.

Sprinkle with paprika. Cover and bake 1 1/4 hours or until chicken is tender. Remove cover and bake another 10 minutes to brown.

NOTE: One serving is an excellent source of fiber.

*Sodium is figured for reduced sodium.

This meal-in-a-pot is great for company. It takes only minutes to assemble and requires no attention while baking.

Makes 5 servings

Each Serving
2 pieces of chicken and 1
   cup of rice/carrots

Carb Servings
3

Exchanges
2 starch
2 vegetable
4 lean meat

Nutrient Analysis
calories 373
total fat 7g
saturated fat 2g
cholesterol 84mg
sodium 350mg
total carbohydrate 43g
dietary fiber 5g
sugars 8g
protein 34g

Using a covered baking pan steams the chicken and results in tender meat cooked in a short period of time. The drippings are thickened to make a delicious gravy. For variety, substitute zucchini and green bell pepper for the carrots.

Makes 4 servings

Each Serving
1/4 recipe

Carb Servings
2 1/2

Exchanges
2 starch
2 vegetable
4 lean meat

Nutrient Analysis
calories 405
total fat 11g
saturated fat 3g
cholesterol 102mg
sodium 197mg
total carbohydrate 39g
dietary fiber 5g
sugars 8g
protein 37g

Roast Chicken and Vegetables

4–5 pounds whole fryer chicken
1 stalk celery, cut into sticks
1/2 onion, quartered
4 small potatoes, not peeled, cut into halves
2 medium carrots, cut into 3" pieces

Optional gravy
drippings, fat removed
unbleached all-purpose flour

Preheat oven to 400 degrees. Prepare chicken by removing giblets and neck and rinsing the entire bird, including cavity. Remove any visible fat. Stuff cavity with celery and onion. Set on a rack in a covered baking pan that has been sprayed with nonstick cooking spray. If using a meat thermometer, insert in breast, without touching the bone. Cover and bake for 30 minutes.

Add potatoes and carrots, being careful not to have them sit in the juices. Cover and cook for 30–45 minutes until chicken is cooked. Chicken is done if the drumstick moves easily. If using a meat thermometer, it should register 190 degrees. Remove skin when carving.

Drain and reserve the liquid. Discard the fat, which will rise to the top. Thicken the liquid for gravy by adding flour. In a covered container, shake 2 tablespoons of flour with 1/4 cup of cold water and add to each 1 cup of reserved liquid. Cook on the stove top or in the microwave, stirring frequently with a wire whisk, until bubbly and thickened.

NOTE: One serving is an excellent source of fiber.

Teriyaki Chicken Breasts

1/3 cup lite soy sauce

1/2 cup water

2 tablespoons brown sugar or the equivalent in artificial sweetener

1 teaspoon ground ginger

1/2 teaspoon garlic powder

1 pound skinless, boneless chicken breasts

Mix the soy sauce, water, sugar, ginger, and garlic powder in a shallow bowl. Add chicken and marinate for 1–2 hours in the refrigerator. Drain chicken and discard marinade.

BARBECUE: Start barbecue. When hot, place chicken on grill. Close hood and cook for 8–10 minutes, turning the chicken halfway through the cooking time. Be sure to cook until chicken is no longer pink.

CONVENTIONAL OVEN: Preheat oven to 350 degrees. Arrange in an 8" × 8" pan that has been sprayed with nonstick cooking spray. Bake for 25–30 minutes until chicken is no longer pink.

BROILER: Preheat broiler. Place chicken on the broiler pan about 3–4 inches from the heat. Broil for 4 minutes. Turn chicken and broil for an additional 4 minutes or until chicken is no longer pink.

The marinade gives a wonderful flavor to this dish. Jumbo shrimp can be substituted for the chicken.

Makes 4 servings

Each Serving
1/4 recipe

Carb Servings
0

Exchanges
3 lean meat

Nutrient Analysis
calories 132
total fat 3g
saturated fat 1g
cholesterol 69mg
sodium 160mg
total carbohydrate 1g
dietary fiber 0g
sugars 1g
protein 25g

You'll find this dish attractive, easy to prepare, and a good choice for company. I use packaged cornflake crumbs in this recipe.

Makes 4 servings

Each Serving
1/4 recipe

Carb Servings
1/2

Exchanges
1/2 starch
3 lean meat

Nutrient Analysis
calories 186
total fat 3g
saturated fat 1g
cholesterol 76mg
sodium 411mg
total carbohydrate 7g
dietary fiber 0g
sugars 2g
protein 31g

Chicken Cordon Bleu

4 skinless, boneless chicken breasts (about 1 pound)
4 thin slices of low-fat ham (about 1/2 ounce each)
2 tablespoons fat-free milk
1/4 cup cornflake crumbs
2 ounces fat-free or reduced-fat Swiss cheese*

Preheat oven to 400 degrees. Cut a pocket in each breast and tuck in one slice of ham. Roll in milk and then cornflake crumbs. Arrange in an 8" × 8" pan that has been sprayed with nonstick cooking spray.

Bake for 25 minutes. Top each breast with 1/2 ounce of cheese and return to oven until cheese is melted.

Using reduced-fat Swiss cheese increases the saturated fat to 2 grams.

Chicken Parmesan

1 cup spaghetti sauce (less than 4 grams of fat
   per 4 ounces), divided
1 pound skinless, boneless chicken breasts
1/2 green bell pepper, sliced
1/2 cup sliced onion
8 ounces fettuccini noodles, uncooked
2 ounces (1/2 cup) grated reduced-fat mozzarella cheese
grated Parmesan cheese (optional)

Spray an 8" × 8" pan or microwave-safe dish with
nonstick cooking spray. Pour 1/2 cup of sauce in the
pan. Place chicken in pan, and top with vegetables and
remaining sauce. Follow directions below for microwave
or conventional oven.

CONVENTIONAL OVEN: Preheat oven to 350 degrees.
Cover with aluminum foil and bake for 30–40 minutes.

MICROWAVE OVEN: Cover, venting the lid, and cook on
high for 10 minutes, depending on thickness of chicken.
Rotate 1/4 turn halfway through cooking.

Top chicken with mozzarella cheese and return to oven,
uncovered, until cheese is melted (conventional oven
about 5 minutes or microwave about 40 seconds).

Meanwhile, prepare noodles according to package
directions, omitting oil and salt. Serve with chicken and
Parmesan cheese (optional).

*This recipe makes a
delicious sauce that tastes
great over noodles.*

Makes 4 servings

Each Serving

Carb Servings
1/2

Exchanges
2 vegetable
3 lean meat

Nutrient Analysis
calories 271
total fat 4g
saturated fat 2g
cholesterol 51mg
sodium 217mg
total carbohydrate 33g
dietary fiber 2g
sugars 4g
protein 25g

This excellent low-fat dish will remind you of Fettuccini Alfredo because it looks and tastes so creamy and rich.

Makes 7 cups
5 servings

Each Serving
1 1/3 cups

Carb Servings
2 1/2

Exchanges
2 1/2 starch
3 lean meat

Nutrient Analysis
calories 316
total fat 7g
saturated fat 1g
cholesterol 54mg
sodium 186mg
total carbohydrate 37g
dietary fiber 2g
sugars 3g
protein 27g

Chicken Dijon Fettuccini

1/4 cup light mayonnaise
1/4 cup fat-free plain yogurt
2 teaspoons Dijon mustard
2 teaspoons dried parsley
8 ounces egg noodles, "no yolk" type (6 cups uncooked)
1 1/2 cups chopped red bell pepper
2 teaspoons chopped garlic
1 pound of skinless, boneless chicken breasts, cut into bite-size pieces

Mix mayonnaise, yogurt, mustard, and parsley to make the sauce. Set aside.

Meanwhile, cook noodles according to package directions, omitting oil and salt. Drain.

Spray a large skillet with nonstick cooking spray and stir-fry pepper, garlic, and chicken until done. Add sauce and noodles and cook on low until heated throughout.

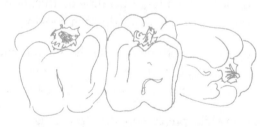

Creamy Chicken Dijon

3 tablespoons light mayonnaise
2 tablespoons fat-free plain yogurt
2 teaspoons Dijon mustard
1 teaspoon honey or the equivalent in artificial sweetener
1 pound skinless, boneless chicken breasts
1 teaspoon dried parsley

Mix mayonnaise, yogurt, mustard, and honey to make the sauce. Set aside. Follow the directions for microwave or conventional oven.

MICROWAVE OVEN: Arrange chicken in a microwave-safe dish that has been sprayed with nonstick cooking spray. Cover, venting the lid, and cook on high for 6–8 minutes, rotating 1/4 turn halfway through cooking time. The time will vary depending on the thickness of the chicken. Drain the liquid, reserving 3 tablespoons. Mix the 3 tablespoons of reserved liquid with the sauce and pour over the chicken. Sprinkle with parsley. Cover and cook for 1–2 minutes or until the chicken is no longer pink and the sauce is heated.

CONVENTIONAL OVEN: Preheat oven to 350 degrees. Arrange chicken in an 8" × 8" pan that has been sprayed with nonstick cooking spray. Bake chicken, covered, for 20 minutes. Drain the liquid, reserving 3 tablespoons. Mix the 3 tablespoons of reserved liquid with the sauce and pour over the chicken. Sprinkle with parsley. Return to oven for 5 minutes or until the chicken is no longer pink and the sauce is heated.

The rich-tasting sauce makes this an extra special chicken recipe. It's a family favorite in my home, and it's definitely a good choice for company.

Makes 4 servings

Each Serving
1/4 recipe

Carb Servings
0

Exchanges
4 lean meat

Nutrient Analysis
calories 174
total fat 6g
saturated fat 1g
cholesterol 69mg
sodium 202mg
total carbohydrate 3g
dietary fiber 0g
sugars 2g
protein 26g

This colorful dish is especially good served with our Spanish Rice and Beans recipe on page 167. Think about following the barbecue method on a hot summer night.

Makes 4 servings

Each Serving
1/4 recipe

Carb Servings
0

Exchanges
3 lean meat

Nutrient Analysis
calories 147
total fat 3g
saturated fat 1g
cholesterol 69mg
sodium 77mg
total carbohydrate 4g
dietary fiber 1g
sugars 2g
protein 26g

Spanish Chicken

1 pound skinless, boneless chicken breasts
3 green onions, chopped
1 cup chopped tomato
1 can (4 ounces) diced green chiles
1/4 teaspoon salt (optional)
1/8 teaspoon ground cumin
1/8 teaspoon ground black pepper

CONVENTIONAL OVEN: Preheat oven to 350 degrees. Spray an 8" × 8" pan with nonstick cooking spray. Arrange chicken in the pan. Top with remaining ingredients. Bake uncovered for 25–35 minutes or until chicken is done.

BARBECUE OR BROILER: Barbecue or broil chicken about 3–4 minutes on each side or until done. Mix remaining ingredients in a microwave-safe bowl. Cover, venting the lid, and cook on high in microwave until heated throughout, about 2 minutes. Pour over cooked chicken.

MICROWAVE OVEN: Arrange chicken in a microwave-safe dish that has been sprayed with nonstick cooking spray. Top with remaining ingredients. Cover, venting the lid, and cook on high for 6–8 minutes, rotating 1/4 turn halfway through cooking time. Time will vary with thickness of chicken.

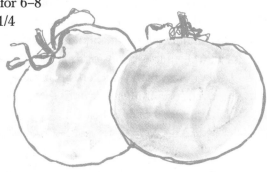

Aloha Chicken

1 can (8 ounces) unsweetened pineapple slices, in juice
1 teaspoon chopped garlic
1 teaspoon cornstarch
1 teaspoon Worcestershire sauce
1 teaspoon Dijon mustard
1/2 teaspoon dried thyme
4 skinless, boneless chicken breasts (1 pound)

Preheat oven to 400 degrees. Drain pineapple, reserving the juice. Combine juice with garlic, cornstarch, Worcestershire, mustard, and thyme.

Arrange chicken in an 8" × 8" pan that has been sprayed with nonstick cooking spray. Pour juice mixture over chicken and bake for 20 minutes. Spoon juices from pan over chicken. Add a pineapple slice to each chicken piece and return to the oven for 5 minutes.

You'll find this to be another good recipe for chicken breasts. The pineapple adds sweetness to this dish.

Makes 4 servings

Each Serving
1/4 recipe

Carb Servings
1/2

Exchanges
1/2 fruit
3 lean meat

Nutrient Analysis
calories 172
total fat 3g
saturated fat 1g
cholesterol 69mg
sodium 104mg
total carbohydrate 10g
dietary fiber 0g
sugars 8g
protein 26g

Seafood

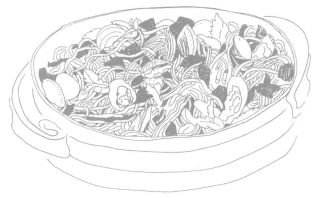

Really fresh fish tastes so good! Even a day or two in the refrigerator makes a big difference in taste. For fresh fish, check the packing date on the label, and try to buy fish packaged on that same day. Then plan on cooking it that evening. Many people don't like fish because they haven't experienced fresh fish. If you can't buy really fresh fish, buy frozen, since it is usually frozen shortly after catching and has a good flavor.

This section presents a number of recipes that give you the choice of using fish fillets, shrimp, and/or scallops. Use different seafoods to provide variety in your diet. The general recommendation is to eat seafood three times a week.

You'll also find additional seafood recipes in the sections "Sandwiches," "Soups and Stews," and "Salads."

Makes 4 servings

Each Serving
1/4 recipe

Carb Servings
0

Exchanges
3 lean meat

Nutrient Analysis
calories 119
total fat 2g
saturated fat 0g
cholesterol 41mg
sodium 127mg
total carbohydrate 2g
dietary fiber 0g
sugars 1g
protein 24g

Barbecued Fish Oriental

1 pound fish fillets
1/4 cup orange juice
1 tablespoon lite soy sauce
2 tablespoons water
2 tablespoons ketchup
1 tablespoon honey or the equivalent
   in artificial sweetener
1 tablespoon dried parsley
1/2 teaspoon ground ginger
1/4 teaspoon ground black pepper

Cut fish into fillets and place a single layer in a shallow
pan. Combine the remaining ingredients, and pour
over the fish. Marinate for 30 minutes to 1 hour in the
refrigerator, turning the fillets once or twice to be sure
they are well coated. Drain and discard marinade.

BROILER: Preheat oven to broil. Spray broiler pan with
nonstick cooking spray. Arrange fish on pan. Broil 2–3"
from heat until done.

BARBECUE: *Before starting the barbecue, spray
aluminum foil with nonstick cooking spray. Place over
rack, poking holes in several areas. Start barbecue. When
ready, place fish on foil, close lid, and barbecue until done.
Allow 10 minutes per inch of thickness.

*Note: Nonstick cooking spray is flammable. Do not spray near open
flame or heated surfaces.*

Curried Sole

1 pound fillets of sole
1/4 cup light mayonnaise
1 teaspoon lemon juice
1 teaspoon curry powder
1 tablespoon dried parsley

Arrange fish in a 9" × 13" baking pan or microwave-safe dish that has been sprayed with nonstick cooking spray. Set aside. Meanwhile, mix mayonnaise, lemon juice, and curry. Spread on fillets. Sprinkle with parsley. Follow directions below for conventional or microwave oven.

CONVENTIONAL OVEN: Preheat oven to 450 degrees. Bake for 4–5 minutes per half-inch thickness of fish or until fish flakes easily with a fork.

MICROWAVE OVEN: Cover, venting the lid, and cook on high for 4–6 minutes, depending on thickness of fish. Rotate dish halfway through cooking.

Curry adds an Eastern touch to traditional baked fish. This is a good dish to serve for company.

Makes 4 servings

Each Serving
1/4 recipe

Carb Servings
0

Exchanges
3 lean meat

Nutrient Analysis
calories 147
total fat 6g
saturated fat 1g
cholesterol 60mg
sodium 193mg
total carbohydrate 2g
dietary fiber 0g
sugars 0g
protein 22g

Makes 4 servings

Each Serving
1/4 recipe

Carb Servings
0

Exchanges
3 lean meat

Nutrient Analysis
calories 135
total fat 4g
saturated fat 1g
cholesterol 42mg
sodium 194mg
total carbohydrate 1g
dietary fiber 0g
sugars 0g
protein 24g

Dijon Fillets

1 pound fish fillets (such as sole or cod)
2 tablespoons light mayonnaise
1 tablespoon Dijon mustard
1 teaspoon lemon juice
1/2 teaspoon paprika

Arrange fish in a 9" × 13" baking pan or microwave-safe dish that has been sprayed with nonstick cooking spray. Mix mayonnaise, mustard, and lemon juice. Spread on fillets. Sprinkle with paprika. Follow directions below for microwave or conventional oven.

CONVENTIONAL OVEN: Preheat oven to 450 degrees. Bake for 4–5 minutes per half-inch thickness of fish or until fish flakes easily with a fork.

MICROWAVE OVEN: Cover, venting the lid, and cook on high for 4–6 minutes, depending on thickness of fish. Rotate dish halfway through cooking.

Fish Poached in Milk

1 pound fish fillets (halibut, snapper, or sole)
1/2 cup fat-free milk
1/4 teaspoon salt (optional)
1/8 teaspoon ground black pepper

Follow directions below for stove top or microwave method.

STOVE TOP: Arrange fish in a large skillet that has been sprayed with nonstick cooking spray. Pour milk over fish and sprinkle with seasonings. Cover and simmer for 1–4 minutes, depending on thickness, or until fish flakes easily with a fork. Remove fish with slotted spatula.

MICROWAVE OVEN: Arrange fish in a microwave-safe dish that has been sprayed with nonstick cooking spray. Pour milk over fish and sprinkle with seasonings. Cover, venting the lid, and cook on high for 4–6 minutes, depending on thickness of fish. Rotate dish halfway through cooking. Remove fish with slotted spatula.

Try this quick method for cooking fish on a busy day.

Makes 4 servings

Each Serving
1/4 recipe

Carb Servings
0

Exchanges
3 lean meat

Nutrient Analysis
calories 118
total fat 2g
saturated fat 0g
cholesterol 42mg
sodium 66mg
total carbohydrate 2g
dietary fiber 0g
sugars 1g
protein 24g

Makes 4 servings

Each Serving
1/4 recipe

Carb Servings
1/2

Exchanges
1/2 starch
3 lean meat

Nutrient Analysis
calories 142
total fat 2g
saturated fat 0g
cholesterol 42mg
sodium 318mg
total carbohydrate 8g
dietary fiber 0g
sugars 0g
protein 24g

Italian Baked Fish

1 pound fish fillets (sole, snapper, or cod)
1/4 cup fat-free Italian salad dressing
1/4 cup cornflake crumbs

Preheat oven to 450 degrees. Marinate fish in dressing for 15 minutes in the refrigerator. Drain, reserving the marinade.

Roll fish in cornflake crumbs. Arrange in a baking pan that has been sprayed with nonstick cooking spray. Drizzle remainder of marinade over fish.

Bake for 4–5 minutes per half-inch thickness of fish or until fish flakes easily with a fork.

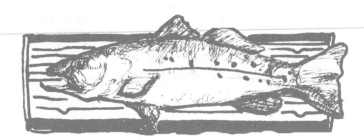

Mushroom-Topped Fillets

1 pound fish fillets (such as sole or cod)
1 tablespoon lemon juice
1/2 cup chopped onion
1 cup sliced fresh mushrooms
1 tablespoon dried parsley
1/4 teaspoon salt (optional)
1/8 teaspoon ground black pepper

Spray a 9" × 13" pan or microwave-safe dish with nonstick cooking spray. Arrange fish in the pan and top with lemon juice. Meanwhile, in a skillet that has been sprayed with nonstick cooking spray, sauté the onions and mushrooms until barely done. Add parsley. Spoon over fish. Season with salt (optional) and pepper. Follow directions below for conventional or microwave oven.

CONVENTIONAL OVEN: Preheat oven to 400 degrees. Bake for 10–15 minutes or until fish flakes easily with a fork.

MICROWAVE OVEN: Cover, venting the lid, and cook on high for 6–8 minutes, depending on thickness of fish. Rotate dish halfway through cooking.

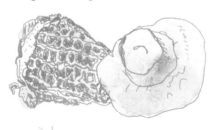

This is a tasty and easy way to prepare fish.

Makes 4 servings

Each Serving
1/4 recipe

Carb Servings
0

Exchanges
3 lean meat

Nutrient Analysis
calories 122
total fat 2g
saturated fat 0g
cholesterol 42mg
sodium 53mg
total carbohydrate 3g
dietary fiber 1g
sugars 1g
protein 24g

This simple recipe has a flavorful breading that adds variety to baked fish.

Makes 4 servings

Each Serving
1/4 recipe

Carb Servings
1/2

Exchanges
1/2 starch
3 lean meat

Nutrient Analysis
calories 164
total fat 4g
saturated fat 1g
cholesterol 65mg
sodium 217mg
total carbohydrate 6g
dietary fiber 0g
sugars 1g
protein 26g

Parmesan Fish Fillets

1/4 cup fine bread crumbs
1/4 cup grated Parmesan cheese
1/2 teaspoon dried thyme
1/4 teaspoon dried basil
1/8 teaspoon onion powder
1/8 teaspoon ground black pepper
1 pound white fish fillets (sole, cod, or snapper)
1/4 cup egg substitute (equal to 1 egg)
4 lemon wedges

Preheat oven to 400 degrees. Combine bread crumbs with Parmesan cheese and seasonings. Mix well.

Dip fish in egg, and then coat with bread crumb mixture. Arrange on a baking sheet that has been sprayed with nonstick cooking spray.

Bake for 10 minutes per inch of thickness, or until fish flakes easily with a fork. Serve with lemon wedges.

Stuffed Fish Fillets

1/2 cup chopped onion
1/2 cup chopped celery
3/4 cup fat-free chicken broth*
3 cups (3 ounces) packaged unseasoned stuffing mix
   (cube type)
1/4 teaspoon dried sage
1/4 teaspoon dried thyme
1 pound fish fillets, such as fillet of sole
paprika, optional

Preheat oven to 350 degrees. In a medium saucepan, combine onion, celery, and broth. Simmer, covered, on low until vegetables are soft. Add stuffing and seasonings. Mix well until blended.

Place a heaping tablespoon of stuffing on each fish fillet. Roll the fillet around the stuffing, and place seam side down in an 8" × 8" pan that has been sprayed with nonstick cooking spray. Sprinkle with paprika.

Bake for 20 minutes or until fish flakes easily with a fork.

Sodium is figured for reduced salt.

This is a unique way to serve fish that is also attractive. The Cheese Sauce on page 78 can be served with this dish. You can also add cooked shrimp to the sauce.

Makes 4 servings

Each Serving
1/4 recipe

Carb Servings
1

Exchanges
1 starch
3 lean meat

Nutrient Analysis
calories 197
total fat 2g
saturated fat 0g
cholesterol 60mg
sodium 281mg
total carbohydrate 19g
dietary fiber 1g
sugars 1g
protein 26g

This is a colorful dish and a good one to prepare with a firm fish such as cod.

Makes 4 servings

Each Serving
1/4 recipe

Carb Servings
1/2

Exchanges
1 vegetable
3 lean meat

Nutrient Analysis
calories 157
total fat 2g
saturated fat 1g
cholesterol 43mg
sodium 277mg
total carbohydrate 8g
dietary fiber 2g
sugars 6g
protein 26g

Zucchini Fish Bake

1 pound firm fish fillets
2 small zucchini, thinly sliced (3 cups)
1 cup spaghetti sauce (less than 4 grams of fat
  per 4 ounces)
1 tablespoon grated Parmesan cheese

Spray a 9" × 13" baking pan or microwave-safe dish with nonstick cooking spray. Arrange fillets in pan. Top with sliced zucchini and spaghetti sauce. Sprinkle with Parmesan cheese. Follow directions below for conventional or microwave oven.

CONVENTIONAL OVEN: Preheat oven to 350 degrees. Cover and bake for 30 minutes or until fish is opaque and flakes easily with a fork. Serve with a slotted spoon.

MICROWAVE OVEN: Cover, venting the lid, and cook on high for 8–12 minutes, depending on thickness of fish. Rotate dish halfway through cooking. Serve with a slotted spoon.

Baked Fish and Rice with Dill Cheese Sauce

1 cup quick-cooking brown rice, uncooked
1 cup boiling water
1 tablespoon dried parsley
1 teaspoon instant chicken bouillon*
1/2 teaspoon Italian seasoning
1 pound fish fillets (such as cod or sole)
1/4 teaspoon paprika

Dill Cheese Sauce

3 tablespoons unbleached all-purpose flour
1 1/2 cups fat-free milk, divided
2 teaspoons dried dill weed
1/8 teaspoon each: ground black pepper and salt
    (optional)
2 ounces (1/2 cup) grated reduced-fat sharp
    cheddar cheese

Preheat oven to 375 degrees. Spray a 9" × 13" baking pan with nonstick cooking spray. Add rice, water, parsley, bouillon, and Italian seasoning. Stir to mix. Cover with aluminum foil and bake for 10 minutes. Top rice with fish fillets. Sprinkle with paprika. Cover and return to oven for 15–20 minutes, until fish is opaque and flakes easily with a fork.

Meanwhile, prepare the sauce by combining the flour with 1/2 cup of milk in a covered container, and shake well to prevent lumps. Pour into a 4-cup glass measuring cup along with the remainder of the milk and seasonings. Cook in the microwave on high for 4–5 minutes, or until bubbly and thickened, stirring with a wire whisk every 60 seconds. Add cheese and stir until melted. Pour over fish before serving.

*Sodium is figured for salt-free.

Here's another easy fish recipe. I especially like the flavor of the dill sauce.

Makes 4 servings

Each Serving
1/4 recipe

Carb Servings
2

Exchanges
2 starch
3 lean meat

Nutrient Analysis
calories 301
total fat 5g
saturated fat 2g
cholesterol 53mg
sodium 242mg
total carbohydrate 27g
dietary fiber 1g
sugars 4g
protein 34g

This is another dish for people who really like curry. Vary or combine seafoods to suit your liking. Serve with rice.

Makes 2 cups
4 servings

Each Serving
1/2 cup

Carb Servings
1/2

Exchanges
1/2 starch
3 lean meat

Nutrient Analysis
calories 145
total fat 2g
saturated fat 0g
cholesterol 42mg
sodium 114mg
total carbohydrate 7g
dietary fiber 1g
sugars 2g
protein 26g

Creamy Curried Seafood

1/2 cup thinly sliced onion
1/2 cup fat-free milk
2 tablespoons unbleached all-purpose flour
1 teaspoon curry powder
1/2 cup fat-free chicken broth*
1 tablespoon dried parsley
1/4 teaspoon salt (optional)
1 pound seafood, such as a firm fish (cod, halibut) cut into bite-size pieces, scallops, and/or shelled and deveined shrimp

Spray a skillet with nonstick cooking spray. Sauté onions until soft.

Meanwhile, combine 1/2 cup milk with flour in covered container, and shake well to prevent lumps.

In the skillet, add curry, flour mixture, broth, and seasonings. Bring to a slow boil, stirring constantly until thickened. Reduce heat, add seafood, and simmer just until seafood is cooked. Serve over rice.

Sodium is figured for reduced salt.

Creamy Seafood Fettuccini

4 ounces egg noodles, "no yolk" type (3 cups uncooked)
1 1/2 cups fat-free milk, divided
1 tablespoon dried parsley
1/2 teaspoon garlic powder
1/4 teaspoon salt (optional)
1/4 teaspoon ground nutmeg
1/8 teaspoon ground black pepper
dash cayenne pepper
1/4 cup grated Parmesan cheese
3 tablespoons sherry, white wine or chicken broth
3 tablespoons unbleached all-purpose flour
1 pound seafood, such as a firm fish (cod, halibut) cut into bite-size pieces, scallops, and/or shelled and deveined shrimp

Cook fettuccini according to package directions, omitting salt and oil. Drain and keep warm.

Meanwhile, spray a skillet with nonstick cooking spray. Pour 1 cup of milk in the skillet and add seasonings, Parmesan cheese, and sherry, wine, or broth. Set over low heat.

Meanwhile, in a covered container, shake flour with remaining 1/2 cup of milk to prevent lumps and add to the skillet. Bring to a slow boil, stirring constantly until thickened. Reduce heat, add seafood, and simmer just until seafood is cooked. Toss with hot fettuccini noodles.

This is a special dish that you will enjoy serving to company or on special occasions. Jumbo shrimp is very good in this recipe as is any combination of seafood. Serve with fresh asparagus.

Makes 4 cups
4 servings

Each Serving
1 cup

Carb Servings
2

Exchanges
2 starch
4 lean meat

Nutrient Analysis
calories 310
total fat 4g
saturated fat 2g
cholesterol 48mg
sodium 217mg
total carbohydrate 32g
dietary fiber 1g
sugars 6g
protein 34g

Makes 6 cups
4 servings

Each Serving
1 1/2 cups

Carb Servings
1

Exchanges
3 vegetable
3 lean meat

Nutrient Analysis
calories 186
total fat 2g
saturated fat 0g
cholesterol 42mg
sodium 438mg
total carbohydrate 15g
dietary fiber 2g
sugars 3g
protein 27g

Seafood Medley

6 ounces fresh snow pea pods (3 cups)
2 cups sliced celery
1 1/2 cups sliced red bell pepper
1/2 cup sliced onion
1 tablespoon lite soy sauce
1/4 teaspoon ground ginger
1/4 teaspoon salt (optional)
2 cups fat-free chicken broth, divided*
3 tablespoons cornstarch
1 pound seafood, such as a firm fish (cod, halibut) cut into
    bite-size pieces, scallops, and/or shelled
    and deveined shrimp

Spray a large skillet with nonstick cooking spray. Add
all ingredients except 1/2 cup of the chicken broth,
cornstarch, and seafood. Simmer, covered, for 5 minutes.

Meanwhile, mix cornstarch with remaining 1/2 cup of
broth. Stir into hot mixture, and heat to a slow
boil, stirring constantly, until thickened.
Reduce heat, add seafood, and simmer just
until seafood is cooked. Do not overcook.
Serve over rice or noodles.

Sodium is figured for reduced sodium.

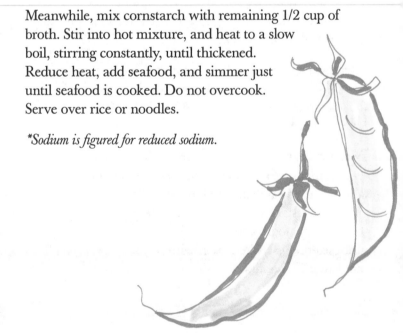

Seafood Pasta

8 ounces ziti pasta, tube shape (3 cups uncooked)
1 tablespoon cornstarch
2 cans (14.5 ounces each) diced tomatoes, not drained*
1 tablespoon chopped garlic
1/2 teaspoon dried oregano
1/4 teaspoon dried basil
1/8 teaspoon ground black pepper
1 pound seafood, such as a firm fish (cod, halibut)
  cut into bite-size pieces, scallops, and/or shelled
  and deveined shrimp
4 ounces (1 cup) grated reduced-fat mozzarella cheese

Preheat oven to 400 degrees. Prepare noodles according to package directions, omitting salt and oil. Drain.

Mix cornstarch with 1/4 cup of the juice from the tomatoes. In a 3-quart saucepan, add cornstarch mixture with the canned tomatoes, garlic, and seasonings. Simmer for 10 minutes, stirring constantly until thickened. Add seafood and simmer until seafood is almost done.

Spray a 9" × 13" pan with nonstick cooking spray. Spread drained noodles in the pan, and top with the seafood sauce. Bake for 10 minutes. Sprinkle cheese on top and return to oven until cheese is melted.

Sodium is figured for no added salt.

I like using ziti noodles in this recipe, but any other noodle would also work. Serve with a tossed salad.

Makes 6 servings

Each Serving
1/6 recipe

Carb Servings
2 1/2

Exchanges
2 starch
1 vegetable
3 lean meat

Nutrient Analysis
calories 301
total fat 5g
saturated fat 2g
cholesterol 38mg
sodium 144mg
total carbohydrate 38g
dietary fiber 2g
sugars 5g
protein 27g

Makes 6 cups
4 servings

Each Serving
1 1/2 cups

Carb Servings
1/2

Exchanges
2 vegetable
3 lean meat
1/2 fat

Nutrient Analysis
calories 211
total fat 7g
saturated fat 1g
cholesterol 42mg
sodium 405mg
total carbohydrate 9g
dietary fiber 3g
sugars 4g
protein 28g

Szechuan Seafood

1 pound seafood, such as a firm fish (cod, halibut)
   cut into bite-size pieces, scallops, and/or shelled
   and deveined shrimp
1/4 cup teriyaki sauce
1 cup sliced red bell pepper
1 cup sliced green bell pepper
2 teaspoons chopped garlic
16 green onions, cut into 1-inch pieces
2–4 tablespoons Szechuan sauce
1/3 cup dry-roasted peanuts, unsalted

Combine seafood with teriyaki sauce, and marinate
at least 1 hour in the refrigerator. Drain and discard
marinade.

Spray a large skillet with nonstick cooking spray and stir-
fry peppers, garlic, and onion until done. Remove from
skillet and keep warm.

Again, spray the skillet with nonstick cooking spray and
stir-fry seafood until done, being careful when turning
fish to prevent flaking. Return vegetables to skillet. Add
remaining ingredients and heat thoroughly.

NOTE: One serving is a good source of
   fiber.

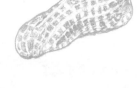

Oriental Seafood

2 cups fat-free chicken broth*
1 tablespoon lite soy sauce
1/2 teaspoon ground ginger
1/4 teaspoon garlic powder
3 ounces coil vermicelli (fine noodles), uncooked
1 medium onion, cut into wedges
1 1/2 cups sliced red bell pepper
1 can (8 ounces) sliced water chestnuts, drained
1/2 cup sliced carrots
1 cup broccoli pieces
1 tablespoon cornstarch
1/4 cup water
1 pound seafood, such as a firm fish (cod, halibut)
    cut into bite-size pieces, scallops, and/or shelled
    and deveined shrimp

Add all but the last three ingredients to a large skillet.
Bring to a boil. Reduce heat to low, cover, and simmer for
8–10 minutes or until vegetables are almost done.

Mix cornstarch with water. Add to skillet and bring to
a slow boil, stirring until thickened. Reduce heat, add
seafood, and simmer just until seafood is cooked.

NOTE: One serving is a good source of fiber.

*Sodium is figured for reduced salt.

*You can make this dish
with jumbo shrimp that
are shelled and deveined.
They are easily found
in the freezer section.
Scallops and halibut are
also very good in this
recipe.*

Makes 7 cups
4 servings

Each Serving
1 3/4 cups

Carb Servings
2

Exchanges
1 1/2 starch
1 vegetable
3 lean meat

Nutrient Analysis
calories 260
total fat 2g
saturated fat 0g
cholesterol 41mg
sodium 368mg
total carbohydrate 31g
dietary fiber 4g
sugars 5g
protein 29g

This excellent low-fat dish will remind you of Fettuccini Alfredo because it looks and tastes so creamy and rich.

Makes 7 cups
5 servings

Each Serving
1 1/3 cups

Carb Servings
2 1/2

Exchanges
2 starch
1 vegetable
3 lean meat

Nutrient Analysis
calories 300
total fat 6g
saturated fat 1g
cholesterol 33mg
sodium 179mg
total carbohydrate 37g
dietary fiber 2g
sugars 3g
protein 25g

Seafood Dijon Fettuccini

1/4 cup light mayonnaise
1/4 cup fat-free plain yogurt
2 teaspoons Dijon mustard
2 teaspoons dried parsley
8 ounces egg noodles, "no yolk" type (6 cups uncooked)
1 1/2 cups chopped red bell pepper
2 teaspoons chopped garlic
1 pound seafood, such as a firm fish (cod, halibut) cut into bite-size pieces, scallops, and/or shelled and deveined shrimp

Mix mayonnaise, yogurt, mustard, and parsley to make the sauce. Set aside. Meanwhile, cook noodles according to package directions, omitting oil and salt. Drain.

Spray a large skillet with nonstick cooking spray and stir-fry the pepper and garlic until done. Remove from skillet and keep warm.

Again, spray the skillet with nonstick cooking spray and stir-fry seafood until done, being careful when turning fish to prevent flaking. Add cooked vegetables, sauce, and noodles. Cook on low until heated throughout.

Pasta with Clam Sauce

1 1/2 pounds fresh steamer clams (about 45 small clams)
3/4 cup chopped onion
1 can (28 ounces) stewed tomatoes, not drained*
1 tablespoon dried parsley
1 1/2 teaspoons chopped garlic
1 1/2 teaspoons dried marjoram
1/4 teaspoon salt (optional)
1/8 teaspoon ground black pepper
1/8 teaspoon crushed red pepper (optional)
6 ounces angel hair pasta, uncooked
grated Parmesan cheese (optional)

Wash and scrub clams. Drain and set aside.

Cook pasta according to package directions, omitting salt and oil. Drain and keep warm.

Add all ingredients, except clams and pasta, to an 8-quart saucepan. Simmer until onion is tender, stirring frequently. Add clams. Cover and cook until clams open, about 7–10 minutes. Transfer pasta to a large serving bowl. Pour clams and sauce over pasta. Serve sprinkled with Parmesan cheese (optional).

NOTE: One serving is a good source of fiber.

*Sodium is figured for no added salt.

This is an attractive way to serve pasta and will appeal to seafood lovers. Mussels can be substituted for clams.

Makes 3 cups pasta plus clams and sauce
4 servings

Each Serving
3/4 cup pasta plus
  1/4 clams and sauce

Carb Servings
3

Exchanges
2 starch
3 vegetable
2 lean meat

Nutrient Analysis
calories 299
total fat 2g
saturated fat 0g
cholesterol 32mg
sodium 84mg
total carbohydrate 46g
dietary fiber 4g
sugars 12g
protein 20g

Makes 3 servings

Each Serving
1/3 recipe

Carb Servings
0

Exchanges
3 lean meat

Nutrient Analysis
calories 133
total fat 2g
saturated fat 0g
cholesterol 56mg
sodium 98mg
total carbohydrate 5g
dietary fiber 0g
sugars 0g
protein 22g

Steamed Clams

2 pounds fresh steamer clams in shells
  (about 60 small clams)
1 cup blush wine
1 medium onion, sliced
2 tablespoons dried parsley
2 teaspoons chopped garlic
1 tomato, chopped (optional)

Rinse and scrub clams. Drain and set aside.

Combine wine, onion, parsley, garlic, tomato, and clams in an 8-quart saucepan. Cover and cook on medium heat for approximately 7–10 minutes or until shells open.

Serve clams in broth and use for dipping.

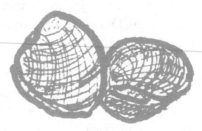

Tuna Patties

1 can (6 ounces) tuna packed in water, drained
2 tablespoons light mayonnaise
1 tablespoon pickle relish
1 teaspoon lemon juice
1 teaspoon dried parsley
1/2 teaspoon onion powder
2 drops Tabasco sauce
3 saltines (unsalted top), crushed

Flake tuna and mix with remaining ingredients. Form into two patties and proceed with one of the methods below.

CONVENTIONAL OVEN: Preheat oven to 350 degrees. Arrange patties on a baking sheet that has been sprayed with nonstick cooking spray. Bake for 25 minutes or until golden brown.

STOVE TOP: Spray a griddle or large skillet with nonstick cooking spray. Cook each patty a few minutes on each side until golden brown.

Serve with a potato and vegetable or as a sandwich on a whole-wheat hamburger bun.

Makes 2 servings

Each Serving
1 patty

Carb Servings
1/2

Exchanges
1/2 starch
3 lean meat

Nutrient Analysis
calories 170
total fat 6g
saturated fat 1g
cholesterol 25mg
sodium 478mg
total carbohydrate 8g
dietary fiber 0g
sugars 3g
protein 22g

This is a good low-fat alternative to traditional tuna noodle casserole. It makes a good luncheon meal, and it is also a good dish to take to a potluck.

Makes 6 cups
8 servings

Each Serving
3/4 cups

Carb Servings
2

Exchanges
2 starch
2 lean meat

Nutrient Analysis
calories 238
total fat 4g
saturated fat 2g
cholesterol 26mg
sodium 273mg
total carbohydrate 30g
dietary fiber 2g
sugars 6g
protein 20g

Tuna Noodle Casserole

1 cup sliced celery
8 ounces rotini noodles, corkscrew shape
   (3 cups uncooked)
2 cups fat-free milk, divided
1/4 cup unbleached all-purpose flour
1 tablespoon dried parsley
1 teaspoon garlic powder
1 teaspoon onion powder
1/2 teaspoon salt (optional)
1/4 teaspoon ground black pepper
1 cup frozen peas
4 ounces (1 cup) grated sharp cheddar cheese
2 cans (6 ounces each) tuna, packed in water, drained

Preheat oven to 350 degrees. Add celery to noodles, and prepare noodles according to package directions, omitting salt and oil. Drain and set aside.

Meanwhile, in a covered container, shake flour with 1 cup milk to prevent lumps. Pour into a 4-cup glass measuring cup along with the rest of the milk and seasonings. Cook in the microwave on high for 3–4 minutes, stirring with a wire whisk every 60 seconds until thickened. Add peas and microwave for 30 seconds. Add cheese and stir until melted.

In a 2-quart covered casserole, mix noodles and celery with cheese sauce and tuna. Bake, covered, for 30 minutes.

Shrimp Burritos

1/3 cup diced red bell pepper
1/3 cup diced green bell pepper
2 tablespoons diced onion
1/2 cup diced tomato
1 teaspoon chopped garlic
1/2 teaspoon dried cilantro
1/2 teaspoon dried basil
1/4 teaspoon ground cumin
1/2 pound cooked (shelled and deveined) bay shrimp
5 whole-wheat tortillas (8 inch)
1/2 cup salsa, thick and chunky
2 ounces (1/2 cup) grated reduced-fat cheddar cheese

Preheat oven to 350 degrees. Spray skillet with nonstick cooking spray. Over medium heat, sauté first three ingredients until tender. Mix in tomato, garlic, and seasonings. Sauté 1–2 minutes. Remove from heat and add shrimp.

Spoon filling onto each tortilla. Roll tightly and place seam side down in an 8" × 8" baking dish that has been sprayed with nonstick cooking spray. Pour salsa over tortillas. Bake 10 minutes. Top with cheese and return to the oven until cheese is melted.

This simple dish will be enjoyed by anyone who likes seafood and Mexican food. Look for the small cooked shrimp in the freezer section.

Makes 5 servings

Each Serving
1 filled tortilla

Carb Servings
2

Exchanges
1 1/2 starch
1 vegetable
2 lean meat

Nutrient Analysis
calories 216
total fat 4g
saturated fat 1g
cholesterol 78mg
sodium 477mg
total carbohydrate 28g
dietary fiber 1g
sugars 4g
protein 17g

Beef and Pork

Too often, I find people who are tired of chicken and fish because that is what they eat all the time. Include beef and pork in your menus to add variety to your diet. Choosing lean cuts, such as top sirloin and tenderloin, and trimming all visible fat makes these healthy choices. Limit beef and pork to three times a week, and keep portions to 3–4 ounces. You'll find additional recipes in the sections "Sandwiches" and "Soups and Stews."

You'll find this to be a favorite for barbecuing. If using wooden skewers, soak them in water first to prevent burning. Chicken, pork, or shrimp can be substituted for beef.

Makes 4 servings

Each Serving
1/4 recipe

Carb Servings
0

Exchanges
3 lean meat

Nutrient Analysis
calories 139
total fat 5g
saturated fat 2g
cholesterol 65mg
sodium 149mg
total carbohydrate 1g
dietary fiber 0g
sugars 1g
protein 22g

Beef Teriyaki

1/3 cup lite soy sauce
1/2 cup water
2 tablespoons brown sugar or the equivalent in artificial sweetener
1 teaspoon ground ginger
1/2 teaspoon garlic powder
1 pound top sirloin, cut into 1" cubes

Mix soy sauce, water, brown sugar, ginger, and garlic powder in a shallow bowl. Add beef and marinate for 1–2 hours in the refrigerator.

Start the barbecue. Drain beef and discard marinade.

Thread beef on skewers, and place on hot grill. Close the hood and cook for 4 minutes. Turn the skewers and cook for another 3–6 minutes or until done to your liking.

Ginger Beef

1 pound top sirloin, sliced thin
1 tablespoon sherry, white wine, or fat-free broth
1 tablespoon water
1 tablespoon lite soy sauce
2 teaspoons granulated sugar or the equivalent
   in artificial sweetener
4 green onions, cut into 1 1/2" pieces
4 slices fresh ginger, 1" × 1 1/2"
1 tablespoon cornstarch
1 cup water

Marinate beef in sherry, water, soy sauce, and sugar
for about 30 minutes in the refrigerator. Drain meat,
reserving the marinade.

Spray a skillet with nonstick cooking spray, and stir-fry
green onions, ginger, and beef until beef is browned. Add
marinade.

Mix cornstarch with water and add to beef. Bring to a
boil, stirring constantly until thickened. Discard ginger
slices. Serve over noodles or rice.

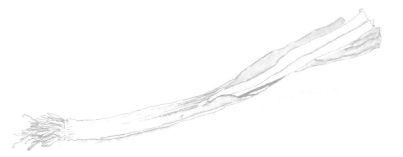

*You'll find this a
pleasant change from
traditional stir-fry
recipes.*

Makes 2 cups
4 servings

Each Serving
1/2 cup

Carb Servings
0

Exchanges
3 lean meat

Nutrient Analysis
calories 157
total fat 5g
saturated fat 2g
cholesterol 65mg
sodium 250mg
total carbohydrate 5g
dietary fiber 0g
sugars 2g
protein 22g

Makes 3 cups
4 servings

Each Serving
3/4 cup

Carb Servings
1/2

Exchanges
1/2 starch
3 lean meat

Nutrient Analysis
calories 187
total fat 5g
saturated fat 2g
cholesterol 65mg
sodium 162mg
total carbohydrate 9g
dietary fiber 1g
sugars 3g
protein 26g

Beef Stroganoff

1 pound top sirloin, cut into strips
1 1/2 cups sliced mushrooms
2 tablespoons unbleached all-purpose flour
1 cup fat-free beef broth*
1 tablespoon dried onion
1 teaspoon chopped garlic
1/4 teaspoon salt (optional)
1/8 teaspoon ground black pepper
1/2 cup fat-free sour cream

Brown meat and mushrooms in a skillet that has been sprayed with nonstick cooking spray.

Combine flour with broth in a covered container, and shake well to prevent lumps. Add to skillet along with onion, garlic, and seasonings. Cook, stirring until thickened and meat is cooked. Add sour cream. Heat but do not boil. Serve over noodles or rice.

Sodium is figured for reduced sodium.

Swiss Steak with Rice

1 pound top sirloin
1 1/4 cups sliced onion
1 1/2 cups sliced green bell pepper
1 cup quick-cooking brown rice, uncooked
2 medium carrots, sliced
1 can (14.5 ounces) diced tomatoes, not drained*
1 2/3 cups fat-free beef broth*
1/2 cup water or red wine
1 teaspoon chopped garlic
1/2 teaspoon dried oregano
1/2 teaspoon dried basil

Preheat oven to 350 degrees. Cut meat into serving pieces.

Spray a 4-quart covered casserole with nonstick cooking spray. Add the meat and the remaining ingredients. Cover and bake for 1 1/2 hours.

NOTE: One serving is a good source of fiber.

Sodium is figured for no added salt/reduced sodium.

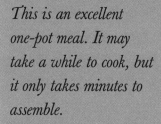

This is an excellent one-pot meal. It may take a while to cook, but it only takes minutes to assemble.

Makes 6 cups
4 servings

Each Serving
1 1/2 cups

Carb Servings
2 1/2

Exchanges
1 1/2 starch
2 vegetable
3 lean meat

Nutrient Analysis
calories 316
total fat 6g
saturated fat 2g
cholesterol 65mg
sodium 243mg
total carbohydrate 36g
dietary fiber 4g
sugars 10g
protein 28g

Serve this great-tasting Chinese dish with rice or low-fat Ramen noodles. If you like spicy-hot dishes, use the larger amount of Szechuan sauce.

Makes 5 cups
5 servings

Each Serving
1 cup

Carb Servings
1/2

Exchanges
2 vegetable
3 lean meat

Nutrient Analysis
calories 199
total fat 9g
saturated fat 2g
cholesterol 52mg
sodium 323mg
total carbohydrate 8g
dietary fiber 2g
sugars 2g
protein 22g

Szechuan Beef

1 pound top sirloin steak
1/4 cup teriyaki sauce
2 teaspoons chopped garlic
1 1/2 cups sliced red bell pepper
3 cups (6 ounces) fresh snow pea pods
10 green onions, cut into 1-inch pieces
2–4 tablespoons Szechuan sauce
1/3 cup dry-roasted peanuts, unsalted

Cut beef into bite-size pieces. Combine with teriyaki sauce and marinate at least 1 hour in the refrigerator. Drain and discard marinade.

Spray a large skillet with nonstick cooking spray and stir-fry beef with garlic for 1–2 minutes. Add remaining ingredients, except peanuts, and stir-fry for 2–3 minutes or until vegetables are tender. Add peanuts.

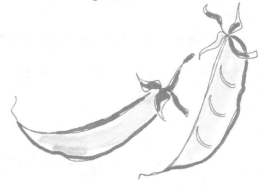

Baked Stuffed Pork Tenderloin

1/2 cup chopped onion
1/2 cup chopped celery
1 1/2 cups fat-free chicken broth*
6 cups (6 ounces) packaged unseasoned
  stuffing mix (cubes)
1/2 teaspoon dried sage
1/2 teaspoon dried thyme
1/8 teaspoon dried marjoram
1 pound pork tenderloin
1 teaspoon dried parsley
1/4 teaspoon salt (optional)
1/8 teaspoon ground black pepper

Preheat oven to 350 degrees. In a large saucepan, combine onion, celery, and broth. Simmer, covered, on low until vegetables are soft. Add stuffing mix, sage, thyme, and marjoram. Mix well until blended. Set aside.

Slice pork into 1/4" slices. Arrange half of the slices in an 8" × 8" pan that has been sprayed with nonstick cooking spray. Top with the stuffing. Place remaining pork slices on stuffing. Sprinkle with remaining seasonings. Cover with aluminum foil. Bake for 30 minutes or until pork is no longer pink.

*Sodium is figured for reduced sodium.

Use packaged stuffing mix in this recipe. It's a simple dish that adds variety to your diet.

Makes 4 servings

Each Serving
1/4 recipe

Carb Servings
2

Exchanges
2 starch
1 vegetable
3 lean meat

Nutrient Analysis
calories 317
total fat 6g
saturated fat 1g
cholesterol 65mg
sodium 411mg
total carbohydrate 35g
dietary fiber 1g
sugars 2g
protein 31g

Makes 7 cups
4 servings

Each Serving
1 3/4 cups

Carb Servings
2

Exchanges
1 starch
3 vegetable
3 lean meat

Nutrient Analysis
calories 285
total fat 5g
saturated fat 2g
cholesterol 65mg
sodium 400mg
total carbohydrate 31g
dietary fiber 3g
sugars 5g
protein 30g

Oriental Pork and Noodles

1 pound pork tenderloin, cut into bite-size pieces
2 cups fat-free chicken broth*
1 tablespoon lite soy sauce
1/2 teaspoon ground ginger
1/4 teaspoon garlic powder
3 ounces uncooked coil vermicelli (fine noodles)
1 medium onion, cut into wedges
1 1/2 cups sliced red bell pepper
1 can (8 ounces) sliced water chestnuts, drained
1/2 cup sliced carrots
1 cup broccoli pieces
1 tablespoon cornstarch
1/4 cup water

Spray a large skillet with nonstick cooking spray, and stir-fry pork until no longer pink. Remove pork and set aside.

Add broth, soy sauce, ginger, garlic powder, coil vermicelli, onion, bell pepper, water chestnuts, carrots, and broccoli to the skillet. Bring to a boil. Reduce heat to low, cover, and simmer for 8–10 minutes or until vegetables are almost done.

Mix cornstarch with water. Add to skillet. Bring to a boil, stirring until thickened. Add pork and heat thoroughly.

NOTE: One serving is a good source of fiber.

Sodium is figured for reduced sodium.

Spicy Pork Burritos

3/4 cup sliced green bell pepper
1/2 pound pork tenderloin, cut into bite-size pieces
2 tablespoons chopped onion
1 teaspoon chopped garlic
1/2 teaspoon dried cilantro
1/2 teaspoon dried basil
1/4 teaspoon ground cumin
1/2 cup diced tomato
2 ounces (1/2 cup) grated reduced-fat cheddar cheese
5 whole-wheat tortillas (8-inch)

Preheat oven to 350 degrees. Spray skillet with nonstick cooking spray. Over medium heat, sauté bell pepper, pork, onion, garlic, cilantro, basil, and cumin until pork is cooked. Mix in tomatoes and cheese.

Spoon filling onto each tortilla. Roll tightly, and place seam side down in an 8" × 8" baking dish that has been sprayed with nonstick cooking spray.

Bake 15 minutes or until heated throughout.

This simple dish will be enjoyed by anyone who likes Mexican food. Salsa can be substituted for the diced tomato.

Makes 5 servings

Each Serving
1 filled tortilla

Carb Servings
2

Exchanges
1 1/2 starch
1 vegetable
2 lean meat

Nutrient Analysis
calories 225
total fat 5g
saturated fat 1g
cholesterol 34mg
sodium 309mg
total carbohydrate 26g
dietary fiber 1g
sugars 4g
protein 18g

Makes 5 cups
5 servings

Each Serving
1 cup

Carb Servings
1 1/2

Exchanges
1 1/2 fruit
2 lean meat

Nutrient Analysis
calories 195
total fat 4g
saturated fat 1g
cholesterol 52mg
sodium 40mg
total carbohydrate 22g
dietary fiber 2g
sugars 12g
protein 19g

Pork with Apples and Grapes

1 pound pork tenderloin, cut into 1/2" cubes
1/2 cup unsweetened apple cider
1 tablespoon brown sugar or the equivalent
  in artificial sweetener
1/2 teaspoon allspice
1/4 teaspoon cinnamon
1 tablespoon cornstarch
1 tablespoon water
2 cups red seedless grapes
2 small apples, not peeled, and cut into slices
  (about 2 cups)

Spray a skillet with nonstick cooking spray. Stir-fry pork until browned. Add cider, sugar, allspice, and cinnamon. Cover and simmer for 5 minutes or until meat is tender.

Meanwhile, mix cornstarch with water and stir into meat mixture. Simmer, stirring constantly, until thickened. Add grapes and apple slices. Cook for 1–2 minutes or just until grapes and apples are heated.

Sweet and Sour Pork

1 pound pork tenderloin, cut into 1/2" cubes

1 teaspoon chopped garlic

1 cup fat-free chicken broth*

1 tablespoon lite soy sauce

1 1/2 cups sliced green bell pepper

2 cups sliced celery

1 can (8 ounces) unsweetened pineapple tidbits, in juice, not drained

2 tablespoons cornstarch

Spray a skillet with nonstick cooking spray. Brown pork with garlic. Add chicken broth, soy sauce, green pepper, and celery. Cover and simmer for 10 minutes.

Meanwhile, drain the pineapple, reserving the juice. Blend cornstarch with reserved pineapple juice and add to the skillet. Cook, stirring constantly, until mixture thickens. Add pineapple and heat thoroughly.

Sodium is figured for reduced sodium.

Serve this with rice or noodles, and you have a complete meal.

Makes 4 cups
4 servings

Each Serving
1 cup

Carb Servings
1

Exchanges
1 fruit
1 vegetable
3 lean meat

Nutrient Analysis
calories 212
total fat 4g
saturated fat 1g
cholesterol 65mg
sodium 339mg
total carbohydrate 18g
dietary fiber 2g
sugars 11g
protein 26g

Ground Meat and Sausage

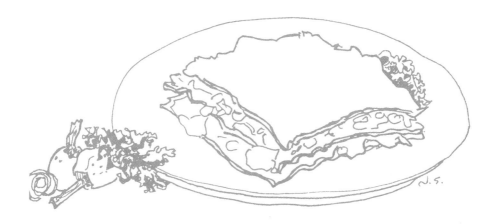

When buying ground beef and ground turkey, look for packages labeled 7% or less fat. If you have trouble finding these, talk to your butcher. Both ground beef and ground turkey work well in the recipes in this section. You'll find additional recipes for ground meat in the sections "Salads" and "Soups and Stews."

If you have not used ground turkey before, you will be pleasantly surprised by the flavor.

Makes 8 cups
8 servings

Each Serving
1 cup

Carb Servings
2

Exchanges
1 1/2 starch
1 vegetable
2 lean meat

Nutrient Analysis
calories 231
total fat 4g
saturated fat 1g
cholesterol 20mg
sodium 587mg
total carbohydrate 30g
dietary fiber 2g
sugars 9g
protein 19g

Italian Baked Ziti

8 ounces ziti pasta, tube shape (3 cups uncooked)
1/2 pound extra-lean ground beef or ground turkey (7% fat)
3 cups spaghetti sauce (less than 4 grams of fat per 4 ounces)
2 cups low-fat cottage cheese
2 tablespoons grated Parmesan cheese
1/4 cup egg substitute (equal to 1 egg)
1 teaspoon dried parsley
1/4 teaspoon garlic powder

Preheat oven to 350 degrees. Cook ziti according to package directions, omitting salt and oil. Drain and set aside.

Meanwhile, crumble meat in a large skillet sprayed with nonstick cooking spray. Sauté until meat is cooked, stirring frequently. Add spaghetti sauce.

Combine cottage cheese, Parmesan cheese, egg substitute, parsley, and garlic powder and mix thoroughly. Add ziti and mix well. Spread 1 cup of spaghetti sauce mixture in bottom of 9" × 13" pan that has been sprayed with nonstick cooking spray. Spoon ziti and cheese mixture into lasagna pan. Pour remaining sauce over ziti and cheese. Cover with aluminum foil and bake 30 minutes.

Pasta Sea Shell Casserole

8 ounces medium-size sea shell pasta (4 cups uncooked)
3/4 pound extra-lean ground beef or
  ground turkey (7% fat)
2 teaspoons chopped garlic
1/2 teaspoon onion powder
3 cups spaghetti sauce
  (less than 4 grams of fat per 4 ounces)
1 tablespoon grated Parmesan cheese (optional)

Prepare pasta according to package directions, omitting salt and oil. Drain and set aside. Meanwhile, continue with either method below.

STOVE TOP: In a large skillet that has been sprayed with nonstick cooking spray, cook meat with garlic and onion powder. Add sauce and heat thoroughly. Add noodles and continue to cook until thoroughly heated. Serve with Parmesan cheese (optional).

MICROWAVE OVEN: In a 3-quart microwave-safe casserole that has been sprayed with nonstick cooking spray, cook meat with garlic and onion powder on high for 3–4 minutes, stirring after each minute to separate the meat. Add sauce and cover, venting the lid, and continue to cook for 3 minutes, stirring halfway through the cooking time. Mix in noodles. Cover, venting the lid, and cook another minute or until thoroughly heated. Serve with Parmesan cheese (optional).

NOTE: One serving is a good source of fiber.

The simplicity of this recipe makes it popular for the working mother. Children and adults alike will enjoy this casserole.

Makes 8 cups
6 servings

Each Serving
1 1/3 cups

Carb Servings
2 1/2

Exchanges
2 starch
2 vegetable
1 lean meat

Nutrient Analysis
calories 270
total fat 5g
saturated fat 1g
cholesterol 35mg
sodium 435mg
total carbohydrate 39g
dietary fiber 3g
sugars 9g
protein 18g

This can be assembled just before cooking, or it can be assembled the day before and refrigerated overnight so it is ready to pop in the oven the next morning.

Makes 6 servings

Each Serving
1/6 recipe

Carb Servings
1

Exchanges
1 starch
2 lean meat

Nutrient Analysis
calories 148
total fat 5g
saturated fat 2g
cholesterol 23mg
sodium 476mg
total carbohydrate 11g
dietary fiber 2g
sugars 4g
protein 13g

Sausage and Egg Casserole

3 slices whole-wheat bread
4 ounces reduced-fat turkey smoked sausage (Polish kielbasa type), chopped
3 ounces (3/4 cup) grated reduced-fat cheddar cheese
1/4 cup sliced green onion or 2 tablespoons chopped dried onion
1 1/2 cups egg substitute (equal to 6 eggs)
1 cup fat-free milk

Preheat oven to 350 degrees. Spray an 8" × 8" pan with nonstick cooking spray. Line pan with bread. Top with sausage, cheese, and onion. Mix eggs with milk and pour over top.

Bake, uncovered, for 40 minutes or until a sharp knife inserted in the center comes out clean.

NOTE: For 12 servings, double this recipe and bake in a 9" × 13" pan for 1 hour.

Macaroni and Sausage Casserole

8 ounces elbow macaroni (2 cups uncooked)
4 cups broccoli pieces
6 ounces of reduced-fat turkey smoked sausage
  (Polish kielbasa type), sliced
1 1/2 cups fat-free milk, divided
3 tablespoons unbleached all-purpose flour
1/4 teaspoon salt (optional)
1/8 teaspoon ground black pepper
4 ounces (1 cup) grated reduced-fat sharp
  cheddar cheese

Prepare macaroni according to package directions, omitting salt and oil. Drain and keep warm.

Meanwhile, add broccoli to a 3-quart microwave-safe casserole dish. Cover, venting the lid, and cook in the microwave on high for 2 minutes. Add turkey smoked sausage and cover, venting the lid. Cook an additional 2 minutes. Keep warm.

Combine 1/2 cup milk with flour in a covered container and shake well to prevent lumps. Pour flour mixture and the rest of the milk into a 4-cup glass measuring cup. Cook in the microwave on high for 4–5 minutes, stirring after each minute with a wire whisk until bubbly and thickened. Add seasonings and cheese.

Add noodles and sauce to the broccoli and mix well. Cook in the microwave for another 30 seconds or until heated throughout.

NOTE: One serving is a good source of fiber.

The addition of low-fat sausage adds variety to traditional macaroni and cheese. It will be a family favorite.

Makes 9 1/2 cups
6 servings

Each Serving
1 1/2 cups

Carb Servings
2 1/2

Exchanges
2 starch
1 vegetable
2 lean meat

Nutrient Analysis
calories 293
total fat 7g
saturated fat 3g
cholesterol 32mg
sodium 468mg
total carbohydrate 37g
dietary fiber 3g
sugars 6g
protein 18g

Makes 8 servings

Each Serving
1/8 recipe

Carb Servings
2

Exchanges
2 starch
1 vegetable
3 lean meat

Nutrient Analysis
calories 305
total fat 7g
saturated fat 2g
cholesterol 41mg
sodium 438mg
total carbohydrate 35g
dietary fiber 3g
sugars 5g
protein 25g

South of the Border Lasagna

1 pound extra-lean ground beef or ground turkey (7% fat)
1 can (14.5 ounces) diced tomatoes, not drained*
1 can (7 ounces) diced green chiles
2 teaspoons chili powder
1 1/2 teaspoons ground cumin
1/2 teaspoon ground black pepper
1/4 teaspoon garlic powder
1/8 teaspoon cayenne pepper
1/4 cup egg substitute (equal to 1 egg)
2 cups low-fat cottage cheese
1 ounce (1/4 cup) grated reduced-fat mozzarella cheese
14 corn tortillas (6 inch)
1 1/3 cups frozen whole kernel corn
2 cups shredded lettuce
1 cup chopped fresh tomatoes
4 green onions, chopped
1 ounce (1/4 cup) grated reduced-fat cheddar cheese

Preheat oven to 350 degrees. Brown meat in a skillet that has been sprayed with nonstick cooking spray. Add canned tomatoes, chiles, and seasonings and set aside.

In a small bowl, combine egg substitute, cottage cheese, and mozzarella cheese.

Spray a 9" × 13" pan with nonstick cooking spray. Cover bottom and sides of pan with 6 tortillas. Layer in this order: corn, 1/2 meat mixture, 4 tortillas, 1/2 meat mixture, 4 tortillas, cheese mixture. Bake for 30 minutes or until bubbly. Remove from oven, and top with remaining ingredients. Serve immediately.

NOTE: One serving is a good source of fiber.

Sodium is figured for no added salt.

Cornbread Casserole

2 cups frozen mixed vegetables
1 pound extra-lean ground beef or ground turkey (7% fat)
1 medium onion, chopped
1 cup fat-free beef broth*
2 tablespoons unbleached all-purpose flour
1 teaspoon chili powder
1/8 teaspoon ground black pepper
1/4 teaspoon salt (optional)

Cornbread Topping:
1/2 cup yellow cornmeal
1/2 cup unbleached all-purpose flour
2 tablespoons granulated sugar
2 teaspoons baking powder
1/4 teaspoon salt (optional)
2 tablespoons canola oil
1/4 cup egg substitute (equal to 1 egg)
1/2 cup fat-free milk

Preheat oven to 350 degrees. Cook frozen vegetables according to package directions, omitting salt. Drain any liquid and set aside. In a skillet that has been sprayed with nonstick cooking spray, brown meat and onion.

Meanwhile, combine flour with broth in a covered container and shake well to prevent lumps. Add to meat mixture along with the chili powder, pepper, and salt (optional). Bring to a boil, stirring constantly, until thickened. Add cooked vegetables and mix well.

Pour into an 8" × 8" pan that has been sprayed with nonstick cooking spray.

In a medium bowl, combine the dry ingredients for the cornbread topping. Add liquid ingredients, and mix just until blended. Spread over meat mixture and bake for 30–35 minutes or until cornbread is golden brown.

NOTE: One serving is a good source of fiber.

Sodium is figured for reduced salt.

You'll find this to be a meal that the whole family will enjoy. Corn can be substituted for the mixed vegetables.

Makes 6 servings

Each Serving
1/6 recipe

Carb Servings
2

Exchanges
2 starch
1 vegetable
2 medium-fat meat

Nutrient Analysis
calories 319
total fat 10g
saturated fat 2g
cholesterol 47mg
sodium 280mg
total carbohydrate 35g
dietary fiber 4g
sugars 8g
protein 22g

If you like cornmeal, you'll like this dish. Homemade chili can be substituted for canned, and it will significantly reduce the sodium. Serve this with coleslaw or a fruit salad.

Makes 6 servings

Each Serving
1/6 recipe

Carb Servings
2 1/2

Exchanges
2 1/2 starch
1 lean meat

Nutrient Analysis
calories 254
total fat 4g
saturated fat 2g
cholesterol 29mg
sodium 572mg
total carbohydrate 39g
dietary fiber 5g
sugars 5g
protein 16g

Chili Tamale Pie

2 1/2 cups water
1 teaspoon salt (optional)
1 1/4 cups yellow cornmeal
2 cans (15 ounces each) reduced-fat turkey chili
   with beans*
2 ounces (1/2 cup) grated reduced-fat cheddar cheese

Preheat oven to 350 degrees. Combine water, salt (optional), and cornmeal in a saucepan. Cook over medium heat, stirring frequently, for about 10 minutes until thick and stiff. Pour into an 8" × 8" baking pan that has been sprayed with nonstick cooking spray. Top with chili and bake for 25 minutes. Sprinkle with cheese, and return to oven for 5 minutes or until cheese is melted.

NOTE: One serving is an excellent source of fiber.

Choose canned chili with less than 30% fat (about 8 grams of fat per 220 calories).

Pasta Olé

6 ounces angel hair pasta, uncooked
1/2 pound extra-lean ground beef or
    ground turkey (7% fat)
1 teaspoon chili powder
1/2 teaspoon paprika
1/2 teaspoon garlic powder
1/2 cup salsa, thick and chunky
1 1/2 cups shredded lettuce
2 ounces (1/2 cup) grated reduced-fat cheddar cheese

Cook noodles according to package directions, omitting salt and oil. Drain and keep warm.

Brown meat in a skillet that has been sprayed with nonstick cooking spray. Add seasonings to meat, and mix well.

Arrange hot noodles on a platter, and top with seasoned meat. Spoon salsa over meat, and top with shredded lettuce and grated cheese. Serve immediately.

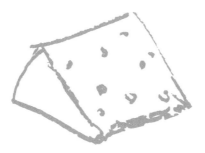

Makes 4 servings

Each Serving
1/4 recipe

Carb Servings
2

Exchanges
2 starch
1 vegetable
2 lean meat

Nutrient Analysis
calories 287
total fat 7g
saturated fat 3g
cholesterol 45mg
sodium 294mg
total carbohydrate 34g
dietary fiber 2g
sugars 2g
protein 21g

This is a family favorite. Serve with salsa and a tossed green salad. The variation, Turkey Enchiladas, is great for using leftover turkey. This recipe can be assembled a day ahead and refrigerated until ready to cook. Increase cooking time to 30 minutes.

Makes 8 servings

Each Serving
1/8 recipe

Carb Servings
2

Exchanges
2 starch
3 lean meat
  —variation, 2

Nutrient Analysis
calories 276
  —variation, 256
total fat 8g
  —variation, 6g
saturated fat 2g
cholesterol 45mg
  —variation, 35mg
sodium 464mg
  —variation, 352mg
total carbohydrate 29g
dietary fiber 2g
sugars 5g
protein 24g
  —variation, 21g

Sour Cream Enchiladas

1/3 cup unbleached all-purpose flour
1 cup fat-free milk
1 1/2 cups fat-free chicken or beef broth*
1 pound extra-lean ground beef or ground turkey (7% fat)
1 1/2 teaspoons ground cumin
1/2 teaspoon chili powder
1/4 teaspoon salt (optional)
1 can (7 ounces) diced green chiles
1/2 cup chopped green onion
1 cup fat-free sour cream
8 whole-wheat tortillas (8 inch)
4 ounces (1 cup) grated reduced-fat cheddar cheese

Preheat oven to 350 degrees. To make the sauce, combine flour with milk in a covered container and shake well to prevent lumps. Pour into a 4-cup glass measuring cup and add the broth. Heat on high in the microwave for 6–7 minutes, stirring every 60 seconds with a wire whisk until bubbly and thickened.

Meanwhile, brown meat in a skillet that has been sprayed with nonstick cooking spray. Add one-half of the sauce to the ground meat along with the seasonings, chiles, green onion, and sour cream.

Spray a 9" × 13" pan with nonstick cooking spray. Fill each tortilla with 1/2 cup of meat sauce and a tablespoon of cheese. Roll and place in pan seam side down. Repeat until all the tortillas are filled. Pour the remaining sauce and any remaining meat mixture over the filled tortillas, being sure that all are covered with sauce. Bake for 20 minutes. Sprinkle with remaining cheese, and return to the oven for 10 minutes.

*Sodium is figured for reduced salt.

VARIATION: *Turkey Enchiladas*–Replace ground meat with 2 cups of cooked, cubed turkey or chicken. Omit the step for browning the meat.

Sweet and Sour Beans

1/2 pound extra-lean ground beef or ground
   turkey (7% fat)
1 medium onion, diced
2 cans (16 ounces each) vegetarian baked beans, drained
1 can (8 ounces) tomato sauce*
2 teaspoons chopped garlic
1 teaspoon Worcestershire sauce
1 teaspoon chili powder
1/2 teaspoon dry mustard
dash of Tabasco sauce
1 can (8 ounces) pineapple tidbits in juice, drained

Spray a skillet with nonstick cooking spray. Brown meat
and onion. Add remaining ingredients and simmer,
uncovered, for 10 minutes.

NOTE: One serving is an excellent source of fiber.

Sodium is figured for reduced sodium.

*Here's a recipe that can
be served as a main dish
or as a side dish. It is
especially good for July
4th parties and will be a
favorite for all ages.*

Makes 4 1/2 cups
9 servings

Each Serving
1/2 cup

Carb Servings
1 1/2

Exchanges
1 starch
1/2 fruit
1 lean meat

Nutrient Analysis
calories 142
total fat 2g
saturated fat 1g
cholesterol 20mg
sodium 166mg
total carbohydrate 21g
dietary fiber 5g
sugars 5g
protein 10g

Makes 8 cups
4 servings

Each Serving
2 cups

Carb Servings**
2

Exchanges**
1 1/2 starch
2 vegetable
3 lean meat
1/2 fat

Nutrient Analysis
calories 336
total fat 10g
saturated fat 3g
cholesterol 71mg
sodium 416mg
total carbohydrate 36g
dietary fiber 6g
sugars 6g
protein 27g

*****Half of the grams of fiber have been subtracted from the grams of total carbohydrate when figuring Carb Servings and Exchanges.*

Unstuffed Cabbage Casserole

1 small head of cabbage (about 1 1/2 pounds)
1 cup boiling water
1 cup quick-cooking brown rice, uncooked
1 pound extra-lean ground beef or ground turkey (7% fat)
1 teaspoon chopped garlic
1/4 teaspoon salt (optional)
1 can (10 3/4 ounces) low-fat condensed tomato soup*
1/2 can water

Preheat oven to 350 degrees. Spray a 2-quart covered casserole with nonstick cooking spray. Add 1 cup of boiling water and rice to the casserole. Cover while preparing the rest of the ingredients.

Slice cabbage. In a large skillet that has been sprayed with nonstick cooking spray, stir-fry cabbage until limp. Add the cabbage to the casserole.

Brown meat with garlic and salt (optional) in the same skillet used to stir-fry the cabbage. Spread over cabbage.

Mix soup with water. Pour over all, and gently stir to mix. Cover and bake for 55 minutes or until rice is cooked and cabbage is tender.

NOTE: One serving is an excellent source of fiber.

Sodium is figured for reduced sodium.

Desserts

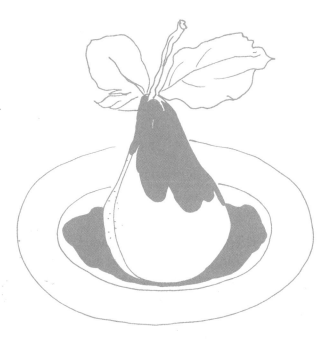

Think of desserts as extras. If you are trying to limit calories, concentrate on eating other foods that will provide more vitamins and minerals. The recipes in this section are lower in calories and fat than most desserts but should still be used in moderation.

Sugar is used in some of the recipes, and these can be used by people with diabetes. However, these foods should be substituted for other carbohydrates and not just added to a meal. Also, as noted on the recipes, artificial sweetener can be substituted for the sugar.

This impressive dessert is perfect for a party and can be prepared in minutes. Serve in a large glass bowl so layers will show. Decorate as you please for the season or holiday.

Makes 8 cups
10 servings

Each Serving
3/4 cup

Carb Servings
1

Exchanges
1 carbohydrate

Nutrient Analysis
calories 105
total fat 0g
saturated fat 0g
cholesterol 2mg
sodium 309mg
total carbohydrate 20g
dietary fiber 0g
sugars 8g
protein 3g

Layered Mousse

1 small box (1 ounce) sugar-free instant white chocolate pudding
1 small box (1 ounce) sugar-free instant chocolate pudding
4 cups fat-free milk
4 cups fat-free whipped topping
Optional decorations for top: fresh fruit (strawberry, cherry, kiwi slice) or shaved chocolate

In a medium bowl, mix white chocolate pudding with 2 cups milk. Stir constantly with a wire whisk for 2 minutes. Refrigerate for 5 minutes.

Meanwhile, in a separate bowl, mix chocolate pudding with 2 cups milk. Stir constantly with a wire whisk for 2 minutes. Refrigerate for 5 minutes.

Keeping the puddings separate, add 2 cups of whipped topping to each bowl, and mix well. Alternately layer mousse in a serving bowl or individual parfait glasses. Decorate as desired.

This is ready to eat, or you can refrigerate it and serve later.

Apple Crisp Parfait

3 cups peeled and sliced apples (about 3 medium apples)
1/3 cup old-fashioned cooking oats
3 tablespoons brown sugar or the equivalent
   in artificial sweetener
2 tablespoons water
1 teaspoon cinnamon

Topping:

4 ounces fat-free vanilla yogurt, sweetened with
   artificial sweetener
1/4 teaspoon cinnamon
1/8 teaspoon ground nutmeg
3/4 cup fat-free whipped topping

Mix apples, oats, brown sugar, water, and cinnamon.
Cook according to microwave or conventional oven
method below.

MICROWAVE OVEN: Pour apple mixture in a 1-quart
microwave-safe bowl. Cover, venting the lid, and cook on
high for 5–7 minutes, rotating 1/4 turn halfway through
cooking time. Depending on thickness of fruit, cooking
time may be longer.

CONVENTIONAL OVEN: Pour apple mixture in a 1-quart
casserole. Bake at 350 degrees for 25 minutes.

TOPPING: Mix yogurt with seasonings. Fold in whipped
topping. Serve a dollop of topping over hot or chilled
apple crisp.

NOTE: One serving is a good source of fiber.

This version of apple crisp takes on a new appearance with a light, flavorful topping.

Makes 2 cups apples and 1 cup topping
4 servings

Each Serving
1/2 cup apples and
   1/4 cup topping

Carb Servings
2

Exchanges
2 carbohydrate

Nutrient Analysis
calories 149
total fat 1g
saturated fat 0g
cholesterol 1mg
sodium 26mg
total carbohydrate 35g
dietary fiber 3g
sugars 24g
protein 2g

This is a low-fat version of a very popular New England dessert. If you like custard, you'll like this recipe. Plan on making this when you're using the oven for a casserole or stew.

Makes 3 cups
6 servings

Each Serving
1/2 cup

Carb Servings
1 1/2

Exchanges
1 1/2 carbohydrate

Nutrient Analysis
calories 126
total fat 0g
saturated fat 0g
cholesterol 2mg
sodium 146mg
total carbohydrate 24g
dietary fiber 1g
sugars 17g
protein 6g

Baked Grape-Nuts Pudding

1/2 cup Grape-Nuts cereal
2 1/2 cups warm fat-free milk
1/2 cup egg substitute (equal to 2 eggs)
1/3 cup granulated sugar or the equivalent in artificial sweetener
1 teaspoon vanilla
1/8 teaspoon salt (optional)
1/2 teaspoon ground nutmeg
fat-free whipped topping (optional)

Preheat oven to 350 degrees. Mix all of the ingredients except nutmeg and whipped topping.

Pour into a 1-quart baking dish that has been sprayed with nonstick cooking spray. Sprinkle with nutmeg.

Bake for 1 hour. Serve with a dollop of fat-free whipped topping (optional).

Raisin Bread Pudding

7 slices of whole-wheat bread, cut into cubes
   (about 4 cups)
1/2 cup seedless raisins
2 cups fat-free milk
3/4 cup egg substitute (equal to 3 eggs)
1/3 cup granulated sugar or the equivalent in
   artificial sweetener
2 teaspoons vanilla extract
1/2 teaspoon cinnamon
1/2 teaspoon ground nutmeg
1/8 teaspoon salt (optional)
fat-free whipped topping (optional)

Preheat oven to 350 degrees. Place bread cubes in an
8" × 8" pan that has been sprayed with nonstick cooking
spray. Mix remaining ingredients, except whipped
topping, and pour over bread cubes.

Bake for 40 minutes or until a sharp knife inserted in
the center comes out clean. Serve with a dollop of fat-free
whipped topping (optional).

NOTE: One serving is a good source of fiber.

VARIATION: *Applesauce Bread Pudding*–Reduce milk to
1 cup, and substitute 1 cup unsweetened applesauce for
the raisins.

NOTE: One serving is a good source of fiber.

*This is a great dessert
that can be assembled in
minutes. Plan on making
when using the oven for
another recipe.*

Makes 9 servings

Each Serving
1/9 recipe

Carb Servings
2
   —variation, 1 1/2

Exchanges
2 carbohydrate
   —variation, 1 1/2

Nutrient Analysis
calories 141
   —variation, 118
total fat 1g
saturated fat 0g
cholesterol 1mg
sodium 200mg
   —variation, 188mg
total carbohydrate 27g
   —variation, 22g
dietary fiber 3g
sugars 19g
   —variation, 16g
protein 6g
   —variation, 5g

Peach Custard

This is a great recipe that uses ripe peaches. Try this for dessert with a dollop of fat-free whipped topping, or serve for breakfast either cold or heated in the microwave.

Makes 9 servings

Each Serving
1/9 recipe

Carb Servings
2

Exchanges
2 carbohydrate

Nutrient Analysis
calories 133
  —variation, 130
total fat 0g
saturated fat 0g
cholesterol 0mg
sodium 46mg
total carbohydrate 29g
  —variation, 28g
dietary fiber 2g
  —variation, 3g
sugars 23g
  —variation, 20g
protein 4g
  —variation, 3g

5 fresh peaches, peeled and sliced (about 5 cups)
1 cup egg substitute (equal to 4 eggs)
1 teaspoon lemon juice
1 teaspoon vanilla extract
1/2 cup granulated sugar or the equivalent
  in artificial sweetener
1/8 teaspoon salt (optional)
1/4 cup unbleached all-purpose flour
1/8 teaspoon cinnamon
fat-free whipped topping (optional)
fresh fruit such as raspberries, strawberries, and
  blueberries (optional)

Preheat oven to 350 degrees. Spread fruit in an 8" × 8" pan that has been sprayed with nonstick cooking spray.

Mix egg substitute, lemon juice, and vanilla extract with an electric mixer or wire whisk. Mix in sugar and salt (optional). Gradually add the flour while whipping to prevent lumps. Pour over fruit. Sprinkle with cinnamon.

Bake for 45 minutes or until a sharp knife inserted in the center comes out clean. Garnish with a dollop of fat-free whipped topping (optional) and fresh fruit (optional).

VARIATION: *Pear Custard*–Substitute fresh pears for the peaches, and mace for the cinnamon.

NOTE: Pear variation—One serving is a good source of fiber.

Baked Pears with Chocolate Sauce

4 small pears with stem intact
2 tablespoons orange juice
4 teaspoons fat-free dark chocolate syrup
  (such as Hershey's)

Peel pears. Partially core from bottom, leaving the stem intact. If necessary, take a small slice off the bottom to make it flat, so the pear can stand without tipping.

Pour orange juice onto a plate, and roll pears in the juice to coat. This will prevent browning.

Arrange pears in a 2-quart microwave-safe casserole. Cover, venting the lid, and cook on high for 3 minutes, rotating 1/4 turn halfway through cooking time. Let sit 5 minutes. Cool in refrigerator until chilled.

To serve, place a pear on a plate with the stem up, and drizzle with chocolate sauce.

NOTE: One serving is an excellent source of fiber.

This is a very attractive dessert that is also delicious. The uniqueness of a pear, including the stem, drizzled with chocolate sauce appeals to all ages. Use pears that are ripe but not too soft.

Makes 4 servings

Each Serving
1 pear

Carb Servings
2

Exchanges
1 fruit
1 carbohydrate

Nutrient Analysis
calories 133
total fat 1g
saturated fat 0g
cholesterol 0mg
sodium 6mg
total carbohydrate 33g
dietary fiber 5g
sugars 20g
protein 1g

Makes 4 cups
4 servings

Each Serving
1 cup

Carb Servings
1

Exchanges
1 fruit

Nutrient Analysis
calories 80
total fat 0g
saturated fat 0g
cholesterol 0mg
sodium 3mg
total carbohydrate 19g
dietary fiber 2g
sugars 10g
protein 1g

Glazed Fruit Cup

1/4 cup sugar-free jam, jelly, or spreadable fruit
4 cups fresh fruit, any combination of berries, grapes, or sliced peaches

Add jelly to a microwave-safe bowl. Cover, venting the lid, and cook on high for about 15 seconds. Cool to room temperature, about 10–15 minutes. Pour over fruit, and gently toss to coat.

Strawberry Yogurt Mousse

1 1/2 cups fat-free whipped topping
8 ounces fat-free strawberry yogurt, sweetened with
   artificial sweetener
2 cups sliced strawberries
4 whole strawberries, optional

Fold whipped topping into yogurt. Add sliced
strawberries. Garnish with a whole
strawberry.

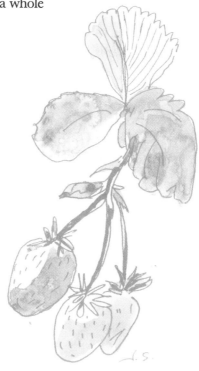

*Serve this light dessert
in parfait glasses with a
fresh strawberry sitting
on top of a dollop of fat-
free whipped topping.*

Makes 4 cups
8 servings

Each Serving
1/2 cup

Carb Servings
1/2

Exchanges
1 1/2 carbohydrate

Nutrient Analysis
calories 45
total fat 0g
saturated fat 0g
cholesterol 1mg
sodium 24mg
total carbohydrate 9g
dietary fiber 1g
sugars 5g
protein 1g

Makes 13 1/2 bars
13 1/2 servings

Each Serving
1 bar

Carb Servings
1

Exchanges
1 fat
1 carbohydrate

Nutrient Analysis
calories 122
total fat 4g
saturated fat 1g
cholesterol 1mg
sodium 300mg
total carbohydrate 18g
dietary fiber 0g
sugars 6g
protein 5g

Chocolate Peanut Butter Frozen Bars

2 packages (1.3 ounces each) sugar-free chocolate
   pudding (cook type or instant)
3 1/3 cups fat-free milk
1/4 cup peanut butter
27 graham cracker squares (2 1/2 inch)

Prepare pudding according to package directions, using only 3 1/3 cups milk. Beat in peanut butter.

Line a 9" × 13" pan with half the graham cracker squares. Three squares will have to be cut in half for all to fit in the pan. Spread pudding mixture over graham crackers. Top with remaining crackers.

Freeze for four hours. Cut into squares and remove from pan. Store in the freezer.

Popsicles

1 package (0.3 ounces) artificially sweetened
   cherry Kool-Aid
1 package (0.3 ounces) sugar-free cherry-flavored gelatin
2 cups boiling water
2 cups cold water

Dissolve Kool-Aid and gelatin in boiling water. Mix in cold water.

Pour into popsicle molds and freeze until firm, about 3–6 hours.

NOTE: Make shaved ice by preparing popsicles as listed above, except pour into a shallow container and freeze until firm (about 3–4 hours). To serve, shave ice by scraping with a spoon.

You can vary the flavor of the gelatin and the Kool-Aid to please everyone in your family.

Makes 16 popsicles

Each Serving
1 popsicle

Carb Servings
0

Exchanges
free

Nutrient Analysis
calories 3
total fat 0g
saturated fat 0g
cholesterol 0mg
sodium 20mg
total carbohydrate 0g
dietary fiber 0g
sugars 0g
protein 1g

Kids will enjoy these fruit popsicles on a hot summer day. Other fruit can be substituted for the peaches.

Makes 8 popsicles

Each Serving
1 popsicle

Carb Servings
1/2

Exchanges
1/2 carbohydrate

Nutrient Analysis
calories 40
total fat 0g
saturated fat 0g
cholesterol 0mg
sodium 3mg
total carbohydrate 10g
dietary fiber 1g
sugars 13g—with artificial
    sweetener 6g
protein 0g

Peach Popsicles

1 can (16 ounces) sliced peaches, in juice, not drained
2 tablespoons granulated sugar or the equivalent in
    artificial sweetener

In a blender, combine all ingredients, and blend until smooth. Pour into popsicle containers or a shallow pan (for shaved ice) and freeze until firm, about 3–5 hours.

Mandarin Yogurt Delight

1 package (0.3 ounces) sugar-free
  orange-flavored gelatin
3/4 cup boiling water
8 ounces fat-free vanilla yogurt, sweetened with
  artificial sweetener
1 can (11 ounces) mandarin oranges, in juice, drained

Dissolve gelatin in boiling water. Add yogurt and stir until smooth.

Chill until the consistency of egg whites, about 20 minutes.

Add drained fruit. Spoon into sherbet dishes and refrigerate until set.

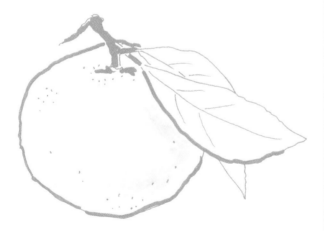

The orange color makes this an attractive dessert. Serve in sherbet dishes with a dollop of fat-free whipped topping. This also works well as a fruit salad.

Makes 2 1/2 cups
5 servings

Each Serving
1/2 cup

Carb Servings
1/2

Exchanges
1/2 carbohydrate

Nutrient Analysis
calories 40
total fat 0g
saturated fat 0g
cholesterol 1mg
sodium 66mg
total carbohydrate 7g
dietary fiber 0g
sugars 5g
protein 3g

You'll enjoy the refreshing taste of this recipe as a salad or as a dessert. This is another great potluck dish and looks especially attractive.

Makes about 5 cups
7 servings

Each Serving
about 3/4 cup

Carb Servings
1

Exchanges
1 fruit

Nutrient Analysis
calories 60
total fat 0g
saturated fat 0g
cholesterol 1mg
sodium 80mg
total carbohydrate 12g
dietary fiber 1g
sugars 9g
protein 3g

Strawberry Delight

1 package (0.3 ounces) sugar-free raspberry-flavored gelatin

1 package (0.3 ounces) sugar-free strawberry-flavored gelatin

1 1/2 cups boiling water

1 package (16 ounces) frozen unsweetened strawberries, sliced

2 cans (8 ounces each) pineapple tidbits, in juice, drained

2 tablespoons lemon juice

8 ounces fat-free vanilla yogurt, sweetened with artificial sweetener

Dissolve gelatin in boiling water. Add strawberries and stir until thawed. Stir in drained pineapple and lemon juice. Pour half into an 8" × 8" glass pan and refrigerate.

Refrigerate the remaining half until the consistency of egg whites.

After about 20 minutes, spread yogurt over the mixture in the 8" × 8" pan. Top with the remaining mixture that is partially set. Chill until firm.

Strawberry-Pineapple Shortcake

1 package (0.3 ounces) sugar-free
  strawberry-flavored gelatin
3/4 cup boiling water
1 package (8 ounces) frozen unsweetened
  strawberries, sliced
2 cans (8 ounces each) crushed pineapple, in juice,
  not drained
1 tablespoon lemon juice
8 slices of angel food cake (about 1 ounce each)

Dissolve gelatin in boiling water. Add strawberries, and
stir until thawed. Stir in undrained pineapple and lemon
juice. Chill.

Top cake slices with chilled sauce.

*You can have shortcake
year-round with this
recipe.*

**Makes 8 cake slices
and 4 cups sauce**
8 servings

Each Serving
1 slice of cake and
  1/2 cup of sauce

Carb Servings
1 1/2

Exchanges
1 1/2 carbohydrate

Nutrient Analysis
calories 113
total fat 0g
saturated fat 0g
cholesterol 0mg
sodium 221mg
total carbohydrate 25g
dietary fiber 1g
sugars 20g
protein 2g

You'll find this pie to be a family favorite.

Makes 7 servings

Each Serving
1/7 pie

Carb Servings
2

Exchanges
2 carbohydrate

Nutrient Analysis
calories 157
total fat 3g
saturated fat 0g
cholesterol 11mg
sodium 127mg
total carbohydrate 29g
dietary fiber 1g
sugars 16g
protein 4g

Banana Cream Pie

1 small package (0.8 ounces) sugar-free vanilla pudding (cook type)
1 2/3 cups fat-free milk
4 ounces fat-free vanilla yogurt, sweetened with artificial sweetener
26 vanilla wafers
2 bananas, about 7" each, sliced (about 2 cups)
1 cup fat-free whipped topping

Prepare pudding according to package directions, except use only 1 2/3 cups of milk. Cool slightly and add the yogurt.

Line the bottom of an 8" pie pan with 12 vanilla wafers (not crushed). Arrange banana slices over the vanilla wafers. Place remaining 14 vanilla wafers standing up around the rim of the pan. Pour in cooled pudding. Top with fat-free whipped topping.

Refrigerate for 2 hours before serving. When serving, cut each piece to include two of the standing-up vanilla wafers.

Chocolate Cream Pie

2 packages (1.3 ounces each) sugar-free chocolate
  pudding (cook type)
3 1/3 cups fat-free milk
33 vanilla wafers
1 cup fat-free whipped topping

Prepare pudding according to package directions, except
use only 3 1/3 cups of milk. Cool.

Line the bottom of a 9" pie pan with 17 vanilla wafers (not
crushed). Place remaining 16 vanilla wafers standing up
around the rim of the pan. Pour in pudding. Top with fat-
free whipped topping.

Refrigerate for 2 hours before serving. When serving,
cut each piece to include two of the standing-up vanilla
wafers.

VARIATION: *Chocolate Peanut Butter Pie*–Add 1/4 cup of
peanut butter to the pudding. This can be served as a
refrigerated or frozen dessert (allow 4–5 hours to freeze).

*This pie is a chocolate
lover's dream. It's almost
too good to be true, yet so
low in fat and sugar!*

Makes 8 servings

Each Serving
1/8 pie

Carb Servings
2

Exchanges
2 carbohydrate
  —variation, 1 fat,
    2 carbohydrate

Nutrient Analysis
calories 156
  —variation, 206
total fat 3g
  —variation, 7g
saturated fat 0g
cholesterol 12mg
sodium 196mg
  —variation, 235 mg
total carbohydrate 27g
  —variation, 29g
dietary fiber 0g
  —variation, 1g
sugars 10g
  —variation, 11g
protein 5g
  —variation, 7g

Makes 8 servings

Each Serving
1/8 pie

Carb Servings
1 1/2

Exchanges
1 fat
2 carbohydrate

Nutrient Analysis
calories 187
total fat 7g
saturated fat 1g
cholesterol 12mg
sodium 221mg
total carbohydrate 25g
dietary fiber 1g
sugars 13g
protein 7g

Chocolate Vanilla Swirl Pie

1 small package (1.3 ounces) sugar-free chocolate pudding (cook type)
3 1/3 cups fat-free milk, divided
1/4 cup peanut butter
1 small package (0.8 ounces) sugar-free vanilla pudding (cook type)
33 vanilla wafers

Prepare chocolate pudding according to package directions, except use only 1 2/3 cups of milk. Beat in peanut butter. Cool.

Prepare vanilla pudding according to package directions, except use only 1 2/3 cups of milk. Cool.

Line the bottom of a 9" pie pan with 17 vanilla wafers (not crushed). Place remaining 16 vanilla wafers standing up around the rim of the pan. Pour in cooled chocolate pudding. Drop in spoonfuls of the vanilla pudding, swirling into the chocolate pudding with the back of a spoon.

Refrigerate for 2 hours before serving. When serving, cut each piece to include two of the standing-up vanilla wafers.

New York Cheesecake

24 ounces fat-free cream cheese (bar type) at
   room temperature
1/2 cup granulated sugar
1/2 teaspoon vanilla extract
1/2 teaspoon almond extract
3/4 cup egg substitute (equal to 3 eggs)
2 tablespoons packaged cornflake crumbs (optional)
2 cups fresh fruit, sliced

Preheat oven to 325 degrees. In a large bowl, combine
cream cheese, sugar, vanilla, and almond extract. Using
an electric mixer, beat at high speed until blended. On low
speed, beat in egg substitute. Increase speed to high, and
continue to beat until well blended.

Spray a 9" pie pan with nonstick cooking spray. Add
cornflake crumbs (optional) to the pan, and shake lightly
to coat the bottom and sides with crumbs. Pour in cream
cheese mixture. Bake for 45 minutes or until center is set
but not firm. Cool on wire rack.

This dessert should be stored in the refrigerator for
several hours before serving. Arrange fresh fruit on top of
cheesecake before serving.

NOTE: Double this recipe for a 9" springform pan,
and bake for 1 hour and 35 minutes. Makes
24 servings. One serving is the same nutritional
value as for 1 serving listed.

Yes, this is a fat-free cheesecake and, yes, it tastes great. Fruit such as blueberries, sliced strawberries, and kiwi can be attractively arranged on top to make this dessert look especially appealing. You can substitute reduced-calorie cherry pie filling for the fresh fruit.

Makes 12 servings

Each Serving
1/12 cheesecake

Carb Servings
1

Exchanges
1 carbohydrate

Nutrient Analysis
calories 94
total fat 0g
saturated fat 0g
cholesterol 10mg
sodium 366 mg
total carbohydrate 14g
dietary fiber 1g
sugars 11g
protein 10g

Serve this fat-free cheesecake during the holiday season. The top will crack, so plan on serving with a dollop of fat-free whipped topping to hide the cracks.

Makes 12 servings

Each Serving
1/12 cheesecake

Carb Servings
1

Exchanges
1 carbohydrate

Nutrient Analysis
calories 86
total fat 0g
saturated fat 0g
cholesterol 10mg
sodium 362mg
total carbohydrate 12g
dietary fiber 0g
sugars 8g
protein 9g

Pumpkin Cheesecake

24 ounces fat-free cream cheese (bar type) at room temperature
3/4 cup canned pumpkin
1/2 cup granulated sugar
1 teaspoon vanilla extract
3/4 cup egg substitute (equal to 3 eggs)
1/2 teaspoon cinnamon
1/4 teaspoon ground cloves
2 tablespoons packaged cornflake crumbs (optional)
fat-fee whipped topping, optional

Preheat oven to 325 degrees. In a large bowl, combine cream cheese, pumpkin, sugar, and vanilla. Using an electric mixer, beat at high speed until blended. On low speed, beat in egg substitute and spices. Increase speed to high, and continue to beat until well blended.

Spray a 9" pie pan with nonstick cooking spray. Add cornflake crumbs (optional) to the pan and shake lightly to coat bottom and sides with crumbs. Pour in cream cheese mixture. Bake for 45 minutes or until center is set but not firm. Cool on wire rack.

This dessert should be stored in the refrigerator for several hours before serving. Top with optional whipped topping when serving.

Duplicate Menus and Grocery Lists

The following pages are copies of the 10 Weeks of Dinner Menus with Grocery Lists from pages 6–25. You can easily remove these from this book to take to the grocery store. Or you can make additional copies and adjust them to meet your needs.

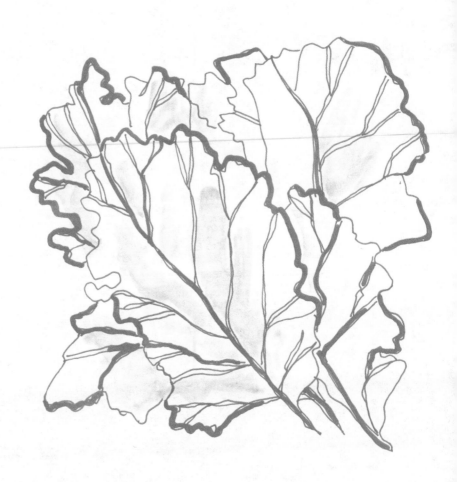

Dinner Menus—Week 1

Ginger Beef • page 249
4 servings
fresh cauliflower* (microwave or steam)
whole-grain roll*

Chicken Parmesan • page 217
6 servings
tossed salad*

Seafood Medley • page 236
4 servings
quick-cooking brown rice*

Taco Salad • page 150
5 servings

Roast Chicken and Vegetables • page 214
4 servings

Week 1—Grocery List

Canned Vegetables, Sauces, & Soups
(To lower sodium, choose no-added-salt or reduced-sodium products.)
chicken broth, fat free (16 oz)
kidney beans (15 oz)
spaghetti sauce (less than 4 g fat
  per 4 oz) 8 oz

Pasta & Rice
fettuccini noodles (8 oz)
quick-cooking brown rice*

Breads & Cereals
whole-grain rolls*

Fresh Produce
green onions (6–8)
onions (1 1/2 medium)
ginger (1 root)
celery (4 stalks)
carrots (2 medium)
red bell pepper (1 1/2 medium)
green bell pepper (1 medium)
snow pea pods, 3 cups (6 oz)
lettuce, 1/2 head (10 oz)
tomatoes (3 medium)
potatoes (4 small)
cauliflower*
salad fixings*

Buy the amount for one meal or substitute a similar food.

Dairy & Cheese
sharp cheddar cheese, reduced fat, grated,
   1 cup (4 oz)
mozzarella cheese, reduced fat, grated,
   1/2 cup (2 oz)
Parmesan cheese, grated (optional)

Meat, Poultry, & Seafood
beef top sirloin (1 lb)
lean ground beef or ground turkey,
   7% fat (1/2 lb)
whole fryer chicken (4–5 lb)
chicken breasts, boneless, skinless (1 lb)
seafood: firm fish (cod, halibut) or scallops,
   and/or shelled and deveined shrimp (1 lb)

Seasonings
ground ginger
chili powder
garlic powder
salt (optional)
ground black pepper

Staples
nonstick cooking spray
lite soy sauce
granulated sugar or artificial sweetener
cornstarch
salad dressing, low fat/fat free of your
   choice*

Miscellaneous
sherry, white wine or fat-free broth (1 Tbsp)
Thousand Island or ranch-style
   dressing (3/4 cup)
tortilla chips, baked (3 oz)

Breakfast foods:

_____

_____

_____

_____

_____

Lunch foods:

_____

_____

_____

_____

_____

Snack foods:

_____

_____

_____

_____

_____

Dinner Menus—Week 2

Curried Sole • page 225
4 servings

Baked Sweet Potatoes or Yams • page 158
4 servings

fresh cooked spinach*
   (microwave or steam)

Patio Chicken and Rice • page 213
5 servings

Spicy Pork Burritos • page 255
5 servings

Waldorf Salad • page 140
6 servings

Venus de Milo Soup • page 112
7 servings

whole-grain roll*

Chicken Dijon Fettuccini • page 218
5 servings

tossed salad*

Week 2—Grocery List

Canned Vegetables, Sauces, & Soups
(To lower sodium, choose no-added-salt or reduced-sodium products.)

chicken broth, fat free (16 oz)
beef broth, fat free (40 oz)
mushrooms, sliced (13 oz)
pimento (2 oz)
stewed tomatoes (14.5 oz)
tomato sauce (8 oz)

Pasta & Rice
quick-cooking brown rice (1 1/2 cups)
orzo or quick-cooking barley (3/4 cup)
egg noodles, "no yolk" type (8 oz)

Breads & Cereals
whole-wheat tortillas, 5 (8-inch)
whole-grain rolls*

Fresh Produce
apples (2 medium)
yams or sweet potatoes (2 medium)
carrots, 4 inch (10 small)
green bell pepper (1 medium)
red bell pepper (2 medium)
tomato (1 small)
celery (2 stalks)
onions (1 large & 1 small)
salad fixings*
spinach*

Dairy & Cheese
milk, fat free (3/4 cup)
yogurt, fat free plain (1/4 cup)
cheddar cheese, reduced fat, grated,
   1/2 cup (2 oz)
Parmesan cheese, grated (1 Tbsp)

*Buy the amount for one meal or substitute a similar food.

Meat, Poultry, & Seafood

chicken breasts, boneless, skinless (1 lb)
chicken (skinless) thighs, legs and breasts
    (8–10 parts)
pork tenderloin, boneless (1/2 lb)
lean ground beef or ground turkey,
    7% fat (1 lb)
fillets of sole (1 lb)

Seasonings

paprika
dried basil
dried cilantro
dried minced onion
dried parsley
ground cumin
curry powder
salt (optional)
ground black pepper

Staples

nonstick cooking spray
cornstarch
fresh or jar of chopped/minced garlic
lemon juice
light mayonnaise (1/2 cup)
Dijon mustard
salad dressing, low fat/fat free of your
    choice*

Miscellaneous

raisins (1/4 cup)

Frozen Foods

mixed vegetables (16 oz)

Breakfast foods:

_____

_____

_____

_____

_____

Lunch foods:

_____

_____

_____

_____

_____

Snack foods:

_____

_____

_____

_____

_____

Dinner Menus—Week 3

Swiss Steak with Rice • page 251
4 servings

Chicken Cordon Bleu • page 216
4 servings

Creamy Mashed
Potatoes • page 160
4 servings

fresh cooked Brussels sprouts*
(microwave or steam)

Oriental Pork and
Noodles • page 254
4 servings

Stuffed Fish Fillets • page 231
4 servings

Cheese Sauce • page 78
1 cup

fresh asparagus* (microwave or steam)

Chicken Chili • page 117
5 servings

raw vegetable slices*

Week 3—Grocery List

Canned Vegetables, Sauces, & Soups
(To lower sodium, choose no-added-salt or reduced-sodium products.)
beef broth, fat free (14 oz)
chicken broth, fat free (22 oz)
tomatoes, diced (29 oz)
water chestnuts, sliced (8 oz)
kidney beans (30 oz)
green chiles, diced (4 oz)

Pasta & Rice
quick-cooking brown rice (1 cup)
coil vermicelli fine noodles (3 oz)

Breads & Cereals
cornflake crumbs (1/4 cup)
unseasoned stuffing mix, cubes
   (3 oz/3 cups)

Fresh Produce
onion (4 medium)
green bell pepper (1 1/2 medium)
red bell pepper (1 1/2 medium)
carrots (3 medium)
potatoes (3 medium)
broccoli, pieces (1 cup)
celery (1 stalk)
asparagus*
Brussels sprouts*
raw vegetable slices*

Dairy & Cheese
milk, fat free (1 1/2 cups)
sour cream, fat free (1/4 cup)
sharp cheddar cheese, reduced fat (2 oz)
Swiss cheese, fat free or reduced fat (2 oz)

Buy the amount for one meal or substitute a similar food.

Meat, Poultry, & Seafood
beef top sirloin (1 lb)
chicken breasts, boneless, skinless (1 1/2 lb)
pork tenderloin, boneless (1 lb)
fish fillets, such as snapper or sole (1 lb)
ham, low fat, 4 slices (1/2 oz each)

Seasonings
dried basil
dried cilantro
dried oregano
dried parsley
dried sage
dried thyme
ground cumin
ground ginger
chili powder
garlic powder
salt (optional)
ground black pepper

Staples
nonstick cooking spray
fresh or jar of chopped/minced garlic
cornstarch
lite soy sauce
unbleached flour

Breakfast foods:

_____

_____

_____

_____

_____

Lunch foods:

_____

_____

_____

_____

_____

Snack foods:

_____

_____

_____

_____

_____

Dinner Menus—Week 4

Beef Stroganoff • page 250
4 servings

fettuccini noodles*
fresh cooked green beans*

Tuna Patties (double recipe) **• page 243**
4 servings

on whole-wheat hamburger buns
with lettuce and tomato slice*

Cucumbers with Dill Yogurt • page 122
4 servings

Garden Minestrone • page 111
6 servings

whole-grain crackers*

Barbecued Fish Oriental • page 224
4 servings

Grilled Eggplant • page 128
4 servings

baked potato*

**Black Bean and Chicken
Casserole • page 209**
5 servings

Citrus Salad • page 136
5 servings

Week 4—Grocery List

Canned Vegetables, Sauces, Soups, & Fish
(To lower sodium, choose no-added-salt or reduced-sodium products.)
beef broth, fat free (56 oz)
chicken broth, fat free (10 oz)
diced tomatoes (14.5 oz)
green beans (14.5 oz)
black beans (15 oz)
green chiles, diced (4 oz)
tuna packed in water (12 oz)

Pasta & Rice
elbow macaroni (1 cup)
quick-cooking brown rice (1 cup)
fettuccini noodles*

Breads, Cereals, & Crackers
whole-wheat hamburger buns (4)

Fresh Produce
grapefruit (1)
orange (1)
cucumber (1 medium)
cabbage, 1/2 small head (5 oz)
carrots (2 medium)
zucchini (1 small)
eggplant (1 lb)
mushrooms, sliced (1 1/2 cups)
salad greens, 1 1/2 quarts (10–12 oz)
red onion (1 small)
green beans*
baking potatoes*
lettuce and tomato slices*

Dairy & Cheese
sour cream, fat free (1/2 cup)
yogurt, fat free, plain (2 Tbsp)
Parmesan cheese, grated (1 Tbsp)
cheddar cheese, reduced fat, grated,
   1/2 cup (2 oz)

Buy the amount for one meal or substitute a similar food.

Meat, Poultry, & Seafood

beef top sirloin (1 lb)
lean ground beef or ground turkey,
    7% fat (1 lb)
fish fillets (1 lb)
chicken breasts, boneless, skinless (1 lb)

Seasonings

dried basil
dried dill weed
dried chopped/minced onion
dried oregano
dried parsley
onion powder
ground cumin
ground ginger
garlic powder
chili powder
cayenne pepper
salt (optional)
ground black pepper

Staples

nonstick cooking spray
lime juice
lemon juice
light mayonnaise
pickle relish
fresh or jar of chopped/minced garlic
Tabasco sauce
lite soy sauce
ketchup
honey or artificial sweetener
cider vinegar
canola oil
olive oil
unbleached flour

Miscellaneous

orange juice (1/4 cup)
saltines, unsalted top (6 individual)
whole-grain crackers*

Breakfast foods:

_____

_____

_____

_____

_____

Lunch foods:

_____

_____

_____

_____

_____

Snack foods:

_____

_____

_____

_____

_____

Dinner Menus—Week 5

Unstuffed Cabbage Casserole • page 270
4 servings

Chicken Caesar Salad • page 151
4 servings

whole-wheat focaccia bread*

Green Chili Pork Stew • page 115
5 servings

Creamy Seafood Fettuccini • page 235
4 servings

fresh cooked broccoli*
 (microwave or steam)

Spanish Chicken • page 220
4 servings

Spicy Spanish Rice • page 168
5 servings

Week 5—Grocery List

Canned Vegetables, Sauces, & Soups
(To lower sodium, choose no-added-salt or reduced-sodium products.)

chicken broth, fat free (8 oz)
tomato soup, low fat, condensed (10.75 oz)
diced tomatoes (14.5 oz)
salsa, thick and chunky (1/3 cup)
green chiles, diced (11 oz)

Pasta & Rice
quick-cooking brown rice (2 1/2 cups)
egg noodles, "no yolk" type (4 oz)

Breads & Cereals
whole-wheat focaccia bread*

Fresh Produce
onion (1 medium)
red onion (1 small)
green onions (3)
celery (1 stalk)
carrots (2 medium)
potatoes (2 medium)
Romaine lettuce, 1 1/2 quarts (12 oz)
cabbage, 1 small head (1 1/2 lb)
tomato (1 medium)
bell pepper (1 medium)
broccoli*

Dairy & Cheese
milk, fat free (1 1/2 cups)
Parmesan cheese (1/3 cup grated)

Buy the amount for one meal or substitute a similar food.

Meat, Poultry, & Seafood
pork tenderloin, boneless (1 lb)
lean ground beef or ground turkey,
   7% fat (1 lb)
chicken breasts, boneless, skinless (2 lb)
seafood: firm fish (cod, halibut) or scallops,
   and/or shelled and deveined shrimp (1 lb)

Seasonings
dried parsley
dried thyme
ground cumin
ground nutmeg
cayenne pepper
garlic powder
salt (optional)
ground black pepper

Staples
nonstick cooking spray
fresh or jar of chopped/minced garlic
cornstarch
unbleached flour

Miscellaneous
Italian or Caesar dressing, fat free or
   reduced fat (1/4 cup)
sherry, white wine or fat-free chicken
   broth (3 Tbsp)

Breakfast foods:

_____

_____

_____

_____

Lunch foods:

_____

_____

_____

_____

Snack foods:

_____

_____

_____

_____

Dinner Menus—Week 6

Oven Beef Stew • page 113
8 servings
orange slices*

Oriental Seafood • page 239
4 servings

Creamy Chicken Dijon • page 219
4 servings
mashed potatoes*
fresh asparagus* (microwave or steam)

Cornbread Casserole • page 265
6 servings
sliced cucumbers*

Hawaiian Chicken Salad • page 153
4 servings
on lettuce leaves*
fresh fruit slices*

Week 6—Grocery List

Canned Fruits & Juices
pineapple tidbits, in juice (16 oz)

Canned Vegetables, Sauces, & Soups
(To lower sodium, choose no-added-salt or reduced-sodium products.)
tomato juice (1 1/2 cups)
water chestnuts, sliced (16 oz)
chicken broth, fat free (2 cups)
beef broth, fat free (1 cup)

Pasta & Rice
coil vermicelli noodles (3 oz)
quick-cooking brown rice (1 1/2 cups)

Fresh Produce
orange slices*
fresh fruit*
onion (3 medium)
celery (3 stalks)
potatoes (2 medium plus enough for mashing for one side dish)
carrots (3 medium)
red bell pepper (2 medium)
broccoli (1 cup pieces)
cucumber*
fresh asparagus*
lettuce leaves*

Dairy & Cheese
egg substitute (1/4 cup, equal to 1 egg)
milk, fat free (3/4 cup)
yogurt, fat free plain (2 Tbsp)

*Buy the amount for one meal or substitute a similar food.

Meat, Poultry, & Seafood
round steak (2 lbs)
lean ground beef or ground turkey,
    7% fat (1 lb)
seafood: firm fish (cod, halibut) or scallops,
    and/or shelled and deveined shrimp (1 lb)
chicken breasts, boneless, skinless (2 lb)

Seasonings
bay leaves
chili powder
curry powder
dried oregano
dried parsley
garlic powder
ground black pepper
ground ginger
salt (optional)

Staples
soy sauce
cornstarch
yellow cornmeal
light mayonnaise
Dijon mustard
honey or artificial sweetener
lemon juice
unbleached flour
granulated sugar
baking powder
canola oil

Frozen Foods
mixed vegetables (2 cups)

Miscellaneous
tapioca (2 Tbsp)

Breakfast foods:

_____

_____

_____

_____

_____

Lunch foods:

_____

_____

_____

_____

_____

Snack foods:

_____

_____

_____

_____

_____

Dinner Menus—Week 7

Italian Curry Pasta • page 192
  4 servings

Mandarin Cottage Salad • page 139
  6 servings

Baked Fish and Rice with
Dill Cheese Sauce • page 233
  4 servings
fresh Brussels sprouts*
  (microwave or steam)

Taco Salad • page 150
  5 servings

Chicken Medley • page 205
  4 servings
whole-wheat roll*

Cheese and Chile
Quesadillas • page 173
  4 servings

Black Bean Soup • page 109
  4 servings

Week 7—Grocery List

Canned Fruits & Juices
mandarin oranges, in juice (11 oz)
pineapple, crushed, in juice (8 oz)

Canned Vegetables, Sauces, & Soups
chicken bouillon, instant (1 tsp)
chicken broth, fat free (2 cups)
beef broth, fat free (1 1/2 cups)
green chiles, diced (4 oz)
black beans (30 oz)
kidney beans (15 oz)
salsa, thick and chunky (1/2 cup)

Pasta & Rice
angel hair pasta (6 oz)
quick-cooking brown rice (1 cup)

Breads & Cereals
whole-wheat tortillas, 4 (8-inch)
whole-wheat rolls*

Fresh Produce
onions (3 medium)
tomatoes (5 medium)
snow pea pods (3 cups)
celery (4 stalks)
red bell pepper (1 large)
lettuce (1/2 head)
green onions (2)
tomatoes (3 medium)
Brussels sprouts*

Dairy & Cheese
Parmesan cheese, grated (2 Tbsp)
cottage cheese, low fat, small curd (2 cups)
sharp cheddar cheese, reduced fat, grated,
  1 1/2 cup (6 oz)
mozzarella cheese, reduced fat, grated,
  1/2 cup (2 oz)

Buy the amount for one meal or substitute a similar food.

yogurt, fat free, vanilla (8 oz)
milk, fat free (1 1/2 cups)

Meat, Poultry, & Seafood
chicken breasts, boneless, skinless (1 lb)
fish fillets, such as cod or sole (1 lb)
lean ground beef or ground turkey,
    7% fat (1/2 lb)

Seasonings
chili powder
dried cilantro
dried dill weed
dried oregano
dried parsley
garlic powder
ground black pepper
ground cumin
ground ginger
Italian seasoning
onion powder
paprika
salt (optional)

Staples
fresh or jar of chopped/minced garlic
unbleached flour
lite soy sauce
cornstarch

Miscellaneous
orange-flavored gelatin, sugar free
    (2 pkgs, 0.3 oz each)
Thousand Island or ranch-style dressing,
    fat free (3/4 cup)
tortilla chips, baked (3 oz)

Frozen
whipped topping, fat free (1 cup)

Breakfast foods:

_____

_____

_____

_____

_____

Lunch foods:

_____

_____

_____

_____

_____

Snack foods:

_____

_____

_____

_____

_____

Dinner Menus—Week 8

Pork with Apples and Grapes • page 256
5 servings

baked sweet potato or yam*
fresh cooked green beans*

Eggplant Parmesan • page 190
4 servings

Bread Sticks • page 99
12 servings

Seafood Dijon Fettuccini • page 240
5 servings

fresh cooked spinach*
(microwave or steam)

Chicken and Stuffing Casserole • page 211
6 servings

fresh cooked broccoli*
(microwave or steam)
whole-berry cranberry sauce*

Creamy Cabbage Soup • page 110
5 servings

rye bread*
sliced fruit*

Week 8—Grocery List

Canned Fruits & Juices
apple cider, unsweetened (1/2 cup)
cranberry sauce, whole berry*

Canned Vegetables, Sauces, & Soups
(To lower sodium, choose no-added-salt or reduced-sodium products.)
spaghetti sauce, less than 4 g fat per 4 oz
   (2 1/2 cups)

Pasta & Rice
egg noodles, "no yolk" type (8 oz)

Breads & Cereals
unseasoned stuffing mix, cubes
   (6 cups/6 oz)
rye bread*

Fresh Produce
apples (2 small)
sliced fruit*
grapes, red seedless (2 cups)
eggplant (1 medium)
red bell pepper (1 large)
cabbage (1 small head)
celery (2 stalks)
onions (2 medium)
green beans*
sweet potato or yam*
fresh spinach*
fresh broccoli*

Dairy & Cheese
mozzarella cheese, reduced fat,
   grated (4 oz)
milk, fat free (3/4 cup)
egg substitute (1/4 cup, equal to 1 egg)

Buy the amount for one meal or substitute a similar food.

Meat, Poultry, & Seafood

pork tenderloin (1 lb)
seafood: firm fish (cod, halibut) or scallops,
    and/or shelled and deveined shrimp (1 lb)
chicken breasts, boneless, skinless (1 lb)
turkey smoked sausage, reduced fat,
    Polish kielbasa type (8 oz)

Seasonings

dried marjoram
dried parsley
dried sage
dried thyme
ground allspice
ground black pepper
ground cinnamon
salt (optional)

Staples

brown sugar or artificial sweetener
cornstarch
light mayonnaise
Dijon mustard
fresh or jar of chopped/minced garlic
unbleached flour

Frozen

whole-wheat bread dough (1 lb)

Breakfast foods:

_____

_____

_____

_____

_____

Lunch foods:

_____

_____

_____

_____

_____

Snack foods:

_____

_____

_____

_____

_____

Dinner Menus—Week 9

Aloha Chicken • page 221
4 servings

acorn or butternut squash*
fresh cooked asparagus*
  (microwave or steam)

Sour Cream Enchiladas • page 268
8 servings

Citrus Salad • page 136
5 servings

Parmesan Fish Fillets • page 230
4 servings

Oven-Fried Parmesan Potatoes • page 161
5 servings

tossed salad*

Beef Hungarian Goulash (v) • page 204
4 servings

Chicken Chop Suey • page 201
4 servings

quick-cooking brown rice*

Week 9—Grocery List

Canned Fruits & Juices
pineapple slices, in juice (8 oz)

Canned Vegetables, Sauces, & Soups
(To lower sodium, choose no-added-salt or reduced-sodium products.)

chicken or beef broth, fat free (1 1/2 cups)
chicken broth, fat free (1 cup)
green chiles, diced (7 oz)
tomatoes, diced (14.5 oz)
tomato sauce (8 oz)
bean sprouts (16 oz or 1 1/2 cups fresh)

Pasta & Rice
ziti pasta (4 1/2 oz)
quick-cooking brown rice*

Breads & Cereals
whole-wheat tortillas, 8 (8-inch)
bread crumbs, fine (1/4 cup)

Fresh Produce
lemon (1)
grapefruit (1)
orange (1)
green bell pepper (1 large)
greens (1 1/2 quarts)
red onion (1 small)
onions (1 large plus 1 medium)
potatoes (4 medium)
celery (3 stalks)
fresh asparagus*
acorn or butternut squash*
tossed salad*

(v) = variation   **Buy the amount for one meal or substitute a similar food.*

Dairy & Cheese
milk, fat free (1 cup)
sour cream, fat free (1 cup)
Parmesan cheese, grated (1/3 cup)
egg substitute (1/4 cup, equal to 1 egg)

Meat, Poultry, & Seafood
chicken breasts, boneless, skinless (2 lb)
white fish fillets, such as sole, cod,
    snapper (1 lb)
lean ground beef or ground turkey,
    7% fat (1 lb)
top sirloin (1 lb)

Seasonings
chili powder
dried basil
dried parsley
dried thyme
garlic powder
ground black pepper
ground cumin
ground ginger
onion powder
paprika
salt (optional)

Staples
fresh or jar of chopped/minced garlic
cornstarch
Worcestershire sauce
Dijon mustard
lime juice
unbleached flour
cider vinegar
canola oil
molasses
lite soy sauce

Breakfast foods:

_____

_____

_____

_____

_____

Lunch foods:

_____

_____

_____

_____

_____

Snack foods:

_____

_____

_____

_____

_____

Dinner Menus—Week 10

Ramen Chicken • page 206
4 servings

Beef and Cabbage Sandwich
(double recipe) • page 177
4 servings
fresh melon slices*

Tuna Patties (double recipe) • page 243
4 servings

Creamy Mashed
Potatoes • page 160
4 servings

Grilled Vegetable
Medley • page 129
4 servings

Skillet Chicken with
Tomatoes • page 207
4 servings

Italian Baked Fish • page 228
4 servings

Black Bean Stuffed
Peppers • page 166
6 servings

Week 10—Grocery List

Canned Vegetables, Sauces, Soups, & Fish
(To lower sodium, choose no-added-salt or reduced-sodium products.)
chicken broth, fat free (4 1/4 cups)
stewed tomatoes (14.5 oz)
black beans (15 oz)
tuna, packed in water (12 oz)

Pasta & Rice
coil vermicelli noodles (4 oz)
quick-cooking brown rice (3/4 cup)

Breads & Cereals
cornflake crumbs (1/4 cup)
pita bread, whole wheat, 2 oz each (4)

Fresh Produce
mushrooms, sliced (1 cup)
carrots (2 medium)
snow pea pods (3 cups)
cabbage (1 small head)
celery (1 stalk)
zucchini (2 small)
red bell pepper (1 medium)
bell peppers, color of your choice
   (3 medium)
potatoes, 6 medium (about 2 lb)
onions (4 medium)
green onions (2)
fresh melon slices*

Dairy & Cheese
milk, fat free (1/4 cup)
sour cream, fat free (1/4 cup)
yogurt, fat free plain (1 cup)
cheddar cheese, reduced fat, grated,
   1/2 cup (2 oz)

Buy the amount for one meal or substitute a similar food.

Meat, Poultry, & Seafood
chicken breasts, boneless, skinless (2 lb)
fish fillets, such as sole, cod, snapper (1 lb)
top sirloin steak (1 lb)

Seasonings
caraway seeds
cayenne pepper
dried oregano
dried parsley
garlic powder
ground black pepper
ground cumin
ground ginger
onion powder
paprika
salt (optional)

Staples
lite soy sauce
cornstarch
Dijon mustard
lemon juice
light mayonnaise
Tabasco sauce
pickle relish
fresh or jar of chopped/minced garlic

Frozen Foods
corn, whole kernel (3/4 cup)

Miscellaneous
saltines, unsalted top (6 crackers)
Italian salad dressing, fat free (1/4 cup)

Breakfast foods:

_____

_____

_____

_____

_____

Lunch foods:

_____

_____

_____

_____

_____

Snack foods:

_____

_____

_____

_____

_____

Index

(v) = *variation*

(v) = *variation*

(*v*) = *variation*

(*v*) = *variation*

(v) = *variation*

(v) = *variation*

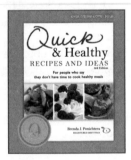
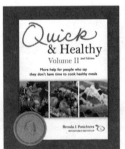
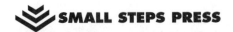